T0303893

Comprehensive Children's Mental Health Services in Schools and Communities

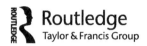
Routledge
Taylor & Francis Group

School-Based Practice in Action Series
Series Editors
Rosemary B. Mennuti, EdD, NCSP
and
Ray W. Christner, PsyD, NCSP
Philadelphia College of Osteopathic Medicine

This series provides school-based practitioners with concise practical guidebooks that are designed to facilitate the implementation of evidence-based programs into school settings, putting the best practices in action.

Published Titles

Assessment and Intervention for Executive Function Difficulties
George McCloskey, Lisa A. Perkins, and Bob Van Divner

Resilient Playgrounds
Beth Doll

Comprehensive Planning for Safe Learning Environments: A School Counselor's Guide to Integrating Physical and Psychological Safety— Prevention through Recovery
Melissa A. Reeves, Linda M. Kanan, and Amy E. Plog

Behavioral Interventions in Schools: A Response-to-Intervention Guidebook
David M. Hulac, Joy Terrell, Odell Vining, and Joshua Bernstein

The Power of Family–School Partnering (FSP): A Practical Guide for School Mental Health Professionals and Educators
Cathy Lines, Gloria Miller, and Amanda Arthur-Stanley

Implementing Response-to-Intervention in Elementary and Secondary Schools: Procedures to Assure Scientific-Based Practices, Second Edition
Matthew K. Burns and Kimberly Gibbons

A Guide to Psychiatric Services in Schools: Understanding Roles, Treatment, and Collaboration
Shawna S. Brent

Comprehensive Children's Mental Health Services in Schools and Communities: A Public Health Problem-Solving Model
Robyn S. Hess, Rick Jay Short, and Cynthia E. Hazel

Forthcoming Titles

Serving the Gifted: Evidence-Based Clinical and Psycho-Educational Practice
Steven I. Pfeiffer

Ecobehavioral Consultation in Schools: Theory and Practice for School Psychologists, Special Educators, and School Counselors
Steven W. Lee

Everyday Program Evaluation for Schools: Implementation and Outcomes
Diane Smallwood and Susan G. Forman

Pediatric School Psychology: Conceptualization, Applications, and Leadership Development
Thomas J. Power and Kathy L. Bradley-Klug

Responsive School Practices to Support Lesbian, Gay, Bisexual, Transgender, and Questioning Students and Families
Emily Fisher and Kelly Kennedy

Comprehensive Children's Mental Health Services in Schools and Communities

A Public Health Problem-Solving Model

Robyn S. Hess ■ Rick Jay Short ■ Cynthia E. Hazel

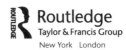

Routledge
Taylor & Francis Group
New York   London

Routledge
Taylor & Francis Group
711 Third Avenue
New York, NY 10017

Routledge
Taylor & Francis Group
27 Church Road
Hove, East Sussex BN3 2FA

Version Date: 20111222

International Standard Book Number: 978-0-415-80448-6 (Hardback) 978-0-415-80449-3 (Paperback)

Library of Congress Cataloging-in-Publication Data

Hess, Robyn.
   Comprehensive children's mental health services in schools and communities : a public health problem-solving model / Robyn S. Hess, Rick Jay Short & Cynthia E. Hazel.
       p. cm.
   Summary: "In this text, the authors propose a public health model for comprehensive children's mental health services that encompasses, rather than replaces, the traditional model in school psychology"-- Provided by publisher.
   Includes bibliographical references and index.
   ISBN 978-0-415-80448-6 (hardback) -- ISBN 978-0-415-80449-3 (paperback)
   1. Child mental health services. I. Short, Rick Jay. II. Hazel, Cynthia E. III. Title.

RJ499.H55 2012
618.92'89--dc23   2011038066

Visit the Taylor & Francis Web site at
http://www.taylorandfrancis.com

and the Routledge Web site at
http://www.routledgementalhealth.com

Contents

SECTION I   Reconceptualizing Our Work

SECTION II   Public Health Problem-Solving Model

SECTION III   From Concept to Action

List of Figures

List of Tables

Series Editors' Foreword

The School-Based Practice in Action series grew out of the coming together of our passion and commitment to the field of education and the needs of children and schools in today's world. We entered the process of developing and editing this series at two different points of our career, although both of us were in phases of transition: one (RWC) moving from the opening act to the main scene and the other (RBM) from main scene to the final act. Despite one of us entering the peak of action and the other leaving it, we both continue to be faced with the same challenges in, and visions for, education and serving children and families.

Significant transformations to the educational system through legislation, such as the No Child Left Behind Act and the reauthorization of Individuals with Disabilities Education Act (IDEA, 2004), have resulted in broad sweeping changes for the practitioners in the educational setting, and these changes will likely continue. It is imperative that as school-based practitioners we maintain a strong knowledge base and adjust our service delivery. To accomplish this, there is a need to understand theory and research, but it is critical that we have resources to move our empirical knowledge into the process of practice. Thus, it is our goal that the books included in the School-Based Practice in Action series truly offer resources for readers to put directly "into action."

To accomplish this, each book in the series will offer information in a practice-friendly manner and will have a companion CD with reproducible and usable materials. Within the text, readers will find a specific icon that will cue them to documents available on the accompanying CD. These resources are designed to have a direct impact on transitioning research and knowledge into the day-to-day functions of school-based practitioners. We recognize that the implementation of programs and the changing of roles come with challenges and barriers, and as such, these may take on various forms depending on the context of the situation and the voice of the practitioner. To that end, the books of the School-Based Practice in Action series may be used in their entirety and present form for a number of practitioners; however, for others, these books will help them find new ways to move toward effective action and new possibilities. No matter which style fits your practice, we hope that these books will influence your work and professional growth.

We are excited to have this innovative book in our series. Hess, Short, and Hazel have brought a public health model of mental health services for children into the schools. This expanded view of comprehensive children's mental health services includes a new role for mental health professionals. The authors offer the background and theory of the use of the model to resolve issues apparent in schools. The procedures for implementing and evaluating programs are clearly explained, and tools such as sample activities, forms, and handouts are provided. It has been a pleasure to work together with Robyn, Rick, and Cynthia to bring you the Public Health Problem-Solving Model to children's mental health service.

Finally, we want to extend our gratitude to Mr. Dana Bliss and Routledge Publishing for their support and vision to develop a book series focused on enriching the practice and service delivery within school settings. Their openness to meeting the needs of school-based practitioners made the School-Based Practice in Action series possible. We hope that you enjoy reading and implementing the materials in this book and the rest of the series as much as we have enjoyed working with the authors on developing these resources.

Rosemary B. Mennuti, EdD, NCSP
Ray W. Christner, PsyD, NCSP
Series Editors, School-Based Practice in Action Series

I

RECONCEPTUALIZING OUR WORK

The significant problems we face cannot be solved at the same level of thinking we were at when we created them.

—**Albert Einstein**

Despite the increased emphasis on a population-based training and service delivery model for school psychology, relatively little has been written to provide guidance concerning how such services might be conceptualized and put into place. This book uses a public health model as the underlying theoretical framework for solving problems and accomplishing goals in schools and communities. We outline and develop a clear, practical procedure, called the Public Health Problem-Solving Model, for implementing and evaluating programs based on public health ideas.

It is often said that change is hard. However, change is also necessary, especially when it comes to addressing the mental health needs of children. Currently, there is a huge imbalance between students' mental health needs and the resources available in schools. Early intervention is more effective than tertiary care. To help organize and focus school psychology practice with respect to addressing the mental health needs of children, we propose adopting a new guiding framework for service delivery. We believe that the field of public health shares many perspectives with school psychology and promotes a broader, population-based focus consistent with the needed new direction of our field.

In Chapter 1, we introduce the public health model and how it compares to a comprehensive model of school psychology services as outlined by the National Association of School Psychologists (NASP). The public health model is both a process of providing services and a philosophy that align with the expansion of school psychology practice, as outlined in recent NASP publications.

In Chapter 2, we outline the continuum of services within a public health model. The three levels of service provision (universal, selective, and indicated prevention) are also compatible with current school psychology practice. However, in a public health model, greater emphasis is placed on health promotion and prevention of disorders. This chapter provides many examples of programs at each level of prevention, as well as a discussion on how to integrate intensive service provision within a prevention framework.

Chapter 3, the last chapter in Section 1, discusses the important groundwork of building collaborations and coalitions. A public health model introduces an approach for addressing systemic needs that cannot be accomplished by any one person. This chapter reviews levels of collaboration and gives guidelines on the key components necessary to build successful partnerships.

One

Intersection of Public Health, Children's Mental Health, and School Psychology

Imagine a pediatric health care system where nobody receives treatment until their physical state is so bad that they are incapacitated. No checkups, no diagnosis or treatment of minor symptoms, no visits to the doctor's office. Symptoms that might indicate a more serious condition are ignored, covered up with a bandage, or dismissed as growing pains or laziness or immaturity. When illnesses are finally diagnosed, they have become so severe and disruptive that patients must be removed from their normal environment and placed in hospitals for intensive care—but only *after* diabetes has been diagnosed or a life-threatening asthma attack has occurred. In this system, insurance companies and caregivers are not concerned about routine wellness checks to monitor growth, there are no vaccines, and families are not informed that these things could be related to problems later on. No education about healthy diet and exercise is provided, and there are no walking trails, fun runs, or nutrition programs. Instead, the only approach is to treat those individuals who demonstrate such advanced and chronic levels of disease that their lives, and those of their families, are disrupted.

In many ways, this scenario describes our present approach to addressing children's mental health needs. Every day, children come to school unable to focus on academics because of family and peer conflict, environmental stressors, and increasing rates of mental health problems. According to a report from the U.S. Department of Health and Human Services (1999), about 20% of children will experience some sort of mental health problem in a given year. Of the children who will receive mental health services, the majority will receive them within the school setting (Burns et al., 1995). As in our example described above, most of these problems will have a significant effect on children's quality of life and educational outcomes but won't be recognized or treated until they become so problematic that they disrupt lives. Children who ultimately exhibit severe educational, behavioral, or emotional difficulties typically receive no formal recognition or help until their problems have forced them into failure.

There is a growing recognition that we cannot provide effective support services by waiting until each child, one child at a time, succumbs to the weight of educational and mental health problems and fails. This recognition has led to the consideration of alternative methods of service delivery. In fact, one of the pervasive themes of the 2001 Conference on the Future of School Psychology was the need for comprehensive, integrated services that promote positive outcomes and prevent problems (Cummings et al., 2004; Dawson et al., 2004). We cannot deal with significant problems of childhood and adolescence by waiting for them to become so severe that lives are disrupted and expensive specialized services are required. We must consider ways in which our schools can foster the adaptive functioning and social-emotional growth of all children. We must develop effective systems for recognizing and dealing with early signs of developing problems as they occur in schools and communities *before* they result in failure and disruption. To do so, we must think about our roles differently and consider how we can create the broadest level of service delivery through our own services and through our collaboration with others (Sheridan & Gutkin, 2000). Systemic approaches such as primary prevention programs and school-community linkages help to ensure that services are provided to all students.

RECONCEPTUALIZING SCHOOL-BASED MENTAL HEALTH SERVICES

Accomplishing this goal will probably require a significant reconceptualization of school psychological services as they relate to children's mental health (Sheridan & Gutkin, 2000). In this book, we propose a reconceptualization of services from the deficit-centric, late-intervention orientation associated with the traditional clinical model to a more systemic, comprehensive perspective that comprises the public health model. Mainstream school psychology presently reflects a variant of the traditional clinical model, wherein services typically are delivered to individual children who have been identified as having a problem. By definition, the problem resides within the child; treatment focuses on changing the child's characteristics to resolve the problem. Although efficient in directing services toward those who need them, this model is reactive and weakness oriented. It fails to recognize and address environmental and systemic contributors to problem behaviors and generally initiates interventions late in the development of these problems.

One approach that holds promise for meeting this difficult goal incorporates a systemic, preventive approach while providing resources to address a broad range of mental health needs. Nastasi (2004) and others have advocated for conceptualizing school mental health from a public health model, specifically, a model in which mental health is considered to be an issue of health and services are directed toward populations rather than individuals. The U.S. Department of Health and Human Services (1999) supports an approach that emphasizes screening of the general population, provides prevention and mental health promotion, increases access to services for all, attends to environmental resources, and evaluates services. A public health model promotes the idea of a continuum of services available to meet the broadest needs, with an emphasis on prevention.

DEFINING PUBLIC HEALTH

When people think of public health, they often consider policies related to clean air and water, or perhaps they envision a dramatic public service announcement or a local campaign encouraging children to wear bike helmets. These examples are part of the services of public health. There is no agreed-upon definition of public health; however, in the document titled *The Future of Public Health* (Institute of Medicine, 1988), public health is defined as "what society does collectively to assure the conditions for people to be healthy" (p. 1). Public health can also be viewed as a social movement. For example, Dan E. Beauchamp (1976), a professor and philosopher on public health, wrote that "public health should be a way of doing justice, a way of asserting the value and priority of all human life" (p. 8).

These broad statements capture one of the key ideas of public health. The focus is on the population rather than the person. When the emphasis is placed on meeting the needs of many rather than a few, change must occur in the environment. Further, a public health model focuses on prevention and promotion of positive outcomes. To best understand where there is a need from a public health-based approach, population-based assessments are carried out. These assessments not only help to pinpoint in which areas intervention is most needed, but they also help to identify the determinants of health. According to Miles, Esperitu, Horen, Sebian, & Waetzig (2010), "determinants are malleable factors that are part of the social, economic, physical, or geographical environment, can be influenced by policies and programs, and contribute to the good and poor health of a population in order to determine which factors, if modified, would lead to positive outcomes" (p. 40).

A public health model also refers to a process for addressing health-related needs within a community. As noted above, assessment is key and is considered a core function in this process. The second core function is policy development. In a school setting, this second component might include both policy development and intervention/prevention implementation. For example, if school leaders decide that a healthy lifestyle program is to be included as part of the broader academic curriculum, that reflects policy development. The programming delivered in each setting (e.g., physical education classes, nutrition awareness programs) is considered the intervention.

The final core function, assurance, refers to the idea that whatever is put in place, the policy and/or the intervention, is actually carried out. This general process should seem familiar; both problem-solving and public health models include efforts to define an issue or a problem, to create an intervention, and to ensure that it has been implemented with fidelity.

Within a public health model, there are also a number of steps within each of these broad core functions or actions that provide further guidance on the process for addressing an issue. These steps are referred to as the Ten Essential Services and define each of these functions in an operationalized manner (Miles et al., 2010). Table 1.1 provides the essential services associated with each core function.

From a public health perspective, prevention planning is accomplished through information and empowerment, the training of caregivers and service providers, coordination of

Table 1.1   Core Functions and Essential Services of Public Health

Core Function: Assessment

1. Monitor health status to identify and solve community health problems.
2. Diagnose and investigate health problems and health hazards in the community.

Core Function: Policy Development

3. Inform, educate, and empower people about health issues.
4. Mobilize community partnerships and action to identify and solve health problems.
5. Develop policies and plans that support individual and community health efforts.

Core Function: Assurance

6. Enforce laws and regulations that protect health and ensure safety.
7. Link people to needed personal health services and assure the provision of health care when otherwise unavailable.
8. Assure a competent public and personal health care workforce.
9. Evaluate effectiveness, accessibility, and quality of personal and population-based health services.
10. Research for new insights and innovative solutions to health problems.

services, and policy and advocacy actions. However, there are other available frameworks that allow us to focus even more broadly in our systemic change efforts. These other frameworks are similar to a public health model in that they outline levels and strategies for building a coalition, empowering stakeholders, and advocating and impacting public policy. Even though these models have been developed and implemented in different contexts (e.g., schools, community), each of them covers similar concepts. We refer interested readers to the works of Cohen and Swift (1999), Dowrick (1998), and Nastasi (2004).

CD Activity 1.1 invites readers to consider their practices and perspectives on children's mental health as related to their own settings.

CURRENT APPROACHES TO ADDRESSING CHILDREN'S MENTAL HEALTH IN THE SCHOOLS

To accompany our new approach, we need to define what we mean by children's mental health. Historically, we have not had a clear vision for what constitutes mental health and instead have defined it as the absence of disorder (Doll & Yoon, 2010). In this work, we have adopted the definition provided in the Surgeon General's Report (U.S. Department of Health and Human Services, 1999) that "child mental health is characterized by achievement of expected developmental cognitive, emotional, and social milestones as well as secure attachments, satisfying social relationships, and effective coping skills" (p. 123). This definition conforms to the comprehensive precepts of diagnosis, prevention, and treatment underlying the broad field of developmental psychopathology (Cichetti, 2010; Drabick & Kendall, 2010; Ialongo et al., 2006).

Within the field of school psychology, we have witnessed a similar shift toward positive approaches rather than simply addressing what is wrong with an individual. As early as the late 1950s, efforts to attend to the positive aspects of human experience within adult populations were beginning. However, it has only been in the past 20 years that concepts such as wellness (Cowen, 1991), primary prevention (Coie et al., 1993), developmental assets (Scales & Leffert, 1999), and positive youth development (Catalano, Berglund, Ryan, Lonczak, & Hawkins, 2004) have focused on children and adolescents. With the publication of a special issue on positive psychology in *American Psychologist* (Seligman & Csikszentmihalyi, 2000), the shift toward ideas of prevention, promotion, and optimizing life experiences have grown exponentially. Although there are subtle differences between primary prevention, wellness, and positive psychology (Cowen & Kilmer, 2002), each of these movements delivers a consistent message: It is no longer sufficient to use a medical model to understand children's mental health.

A public health model, which emphasizes prevention, promotion of positive outcomes, population-based assessment and interventions, and comprehensive services, may provide a better paradigm for children's mental health services in the schools. The public health model defines issues and clinical problems as being multi-determined and existing along a developmental spectrum. Effective public health interventions rely on careful diagnosis of system problems and focus treatment on important individual, family, school, and community targets. Rather than replacing the traditional clinical model, the public health model broadens the scope and definition of children's mental health services to include a full continuum of service provision.

APPLYING A PUBLIC HEALTH MODEL TO THE PRACTICE OF SCHOOL PSYCHOLOGY

Although the language used to define these services is different than what is familiar to school psychology practice, it is easy to see the areas of overlap. Public health conceptualizations of school-based practice are evident in *School Psychology: A Blueprint for Training and Practice III [Blueprint III]* (Ysseldyke et al., 2006). As in previous versions, the latest document outlines a set of competency domains that underlie school psychology; it also adds several new domains, including "Systems Thinking" and "Wellness, Mental Health, & Development of Life Competencies," which clearly reflect movement toward population-based conceptualizations of practice. Further, *Blueprint III* was organized to reflect a continuum of services, ranging from universal delivery (assessment of and intervention with populations to improve functioning or prevent problems) to intensive services (assessment of and intervention with individuals or small groups that exhibit clear problems).

Indeed, Ysseldyke and his colleagues (2006) proposed that the dual goals of school psychologists were to (1) improve competencies for all children, and (2) build and maintain the capacities of systems to meet the needs of all children, suggesting that traditional problem-based individual services should be superseded by systemic, population-based conceptualizations of training and practice. In support of this conclusion, the authors stated, "If the goals of school psychology are to improve competencies for children and build and maintain systems capacity, then the logical next question is: What is the mechanism by which these goals can be attained?" (Ysseldyke et al., 2008, p. 44). *Blueprint III* depicts a service delivery system characterized by variably intensive interventions depending on the severity of student need. Without a doubt, school psychology is evolving from its clinical roots to a broader, more comprehensive specialty, as shown in Figure 1.1.

This blueprint helped to create the foundation for the new revision in the standards for school psychology practice and training. In their revision of practice standards, the National Association of School Psychologists (NASP; 2010) outlined 10 competency domains, which serve as a foundation for how school psychologists should organize and evaluate their practice. The competency domains are organized into three broad dimensions of practice and training: Practices that Permeate All Aspects of Service Delivery; Direct and Indirect Services for Children, Families, and Schools (further divided into Student-Level Services and System-Level Services); and Foundations of School Psychological Service Delivery. Competency domains in the NASP standards are presented in Table 1.2.

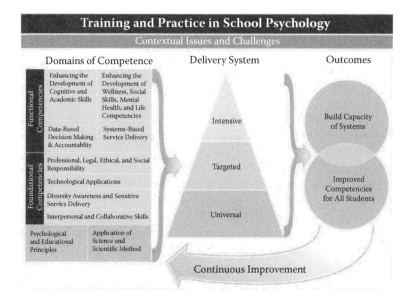

Figure 1.1   Blueprint for training and practice model. (Copyright 2010 by the National Association of School Psychologists, Bethesda, MD. Reprinted with permission of the publisher. www.nasponline.org)

NASP has also provided a graphic representation of these components (see Figure 1.2) that illustrates their relationship in practice. In this model, two aspects of service delivery—data-based decision-making and consultation and collaboration—are key to the delivery of services. There is a continual feedback loop in which the outcomes of services drive additional decision-making and collaborative efforts. Underlying all aspects of these professional services are competencies related to meeting the needs of diverse populations, conducting ongoing research and program evaluation, and functioning in a legal and ethical manner (NASP, 2010).

Many of these competencies align with the Essential Services presented as part of the public health model. For example, one of the 10 competency domains outlined by NASP is data-based decision-making, which is similar to two of the Essential Services which describe monitoring health status and diagnosing problems as the first two services (see Table 1.1). In the traditional school psychology model focusing on services to individuals and small groups, data-based decision-making typically refers to individual assessment and diagnosis. In the public health model, however, a school psychologist might exhibit competency within the same domain by performing a needs assessment within the school to determine areas of strength and concern, and subsequently help to develop school-wide programming to address identified needs. The target of these efforts would focus on assessment and diagnosis of the school or community population rather than on individual students or small groups of students. Similar parallels can be drawn for consultation, home–school linkages, and program evaluation, as well as other dimensions of competence in school psychology. A comparative table (Table 10.1) is provided in Chapter 10.

The new practice model, titled the *Model for Comprehensive and Integrated School Psychological Services* (NASP, 2010), provides a framework for service delivery. One of the goals of this model, also called the NASP Practice Model, is to support more consistent practice between school psychology practitioners across different states, districts, and schools. For schools that adopt this model, the document advocates for a lower recommended ratio of school psychologists per students than previously. The new ratio, 1:500–700, is thought to provide school psychologists the opportunity to become more involved at different levels of service delivery. We believe that this model aligns well with a public health model, and by integrating the two approaches, school psychologists will be able to better meet the needs of students, families, schools, and communities through comprehensive, preventive programming that is developed and implemented in collaboration with others.

CONCLUSION

Reconceptualizing school psychology services through a public health lens is aligned with the NASP competence domains and training and practice guidelines. It is also in keeping with students' needs and what the public wants for our students: comprehensive mental health supports that assist all students in meeting their academic potential. In the subsequent chapters of this book, we present in detail the components of the public health model applied to the practice of psychology in the school, relate those components to comprehensive children's mental health services, and provide practical examples of school psychological services within the model. Finally, we address new roles for school psychologists, focusing on prevention and promotion, that will likely accrue to our identification with the public health model.

Table 1.2 NASP Competency Domains (NASP, 2010)

Practices That Permeate All Aspects of Service Delivery

Data-Based Decision-Making and Accountability

School psychologists have knowledge of varied models and methods of assessment and data collection methods for identifying strengths and needs, developing effective services and programs, and measuring progress and outcomes. As part of a systematic and comprehensive process of effective decision-making and problem-solving that permeates all aspects of service delivery, school psychologists demonstrate skills to use psychological and educational assessment, data collection strategies, and technology resources, and apply results to design, implement, and evaluate response to services and programs.

Consultation and Collaboration

School psychologists have knowledge of varied models and strategies of consultation, collaboration, and communication applicable to individuals, families, groups, and systems, and methods to promote effective implementation of services. As part of a systematic and comprehensive process of effective decision-making and problem-solving that permeates all aspects of service delivery, school psychologists demonstrate skills to consult, collaborate, and communicate effectively with others.

Direct and Indirect Services for Children, Families, and Schools

Student-Level Services

Interventions and Instructional Support to Develop Academic Skills

School psychologists have knowledge of biological, cultural, and social influences on academic skills; human learning, cognitive, and developmental processes; and evidence-based curricula and instructional strategies. School psychologists, in collaboration with others, demonstrate skills to use assessment and data collection methods and to implement and evaluate services that support cognitive and academic skills.

Interventions and Mental Health Services to Develop Social and Life Skills

School psychologists have knowledge of biological, cultural, developmental, and social influences on behavior and mental health, behavioral and emotional impacts on learning and life skills, and evidence-based strategies to promote social–emotional functioning and mental health. School psychologists, in collaboration with others, demonstrate skills to use assessment and data-collection methods and to implement and evaluate services that support socialization, learning, and mental health.

Systems-Level Services

School-Wide Practices to Promote Learning

School psychologists have knowledge of school and systems structure, organization, and theory; general and special education; technology resources; and evidence-based school practices that promote learning and mental health. School psychologists, in collaboration with others, demonstrate skills to develop and implement practices and strategies to create and maintain effective and supportive learning environments for children and others.

Table 1.2 (continued) NASP Competency Domains (NASP, 2010)

Preventive and Responsive Services

School psychologists have knowledge of principles and research related to resilience and risk factors in learning and mental health, services in schools and communities to support multi-tiered prevention, and evidence-based strategies for effective crisis response. School psychologists, in collaboration with others, demonstrate skills to promote services that enhance learning, mental health, safety, and physical well-being through protective and adaptive factors and to implement effective crisis preparation, response, and recovery.

Family-School Collaboration Services

School psychologists have knowledge of principles and research related to family systems, strengths, needs, and culture; evidence-based strategies to support family influences on children's learning and mental health; and strategies to develop collaboration between families and schools. School psychologists, in collaboration with others, demonstrate skills to design, implement, and evaluate services that respond to culture and context and facilitate family and school partnerships and interactions with community agencies for enhancement of academic and social–behavioral outcomes for children.

Foundations of School Psychological Service Delivery

Diversity in Development and Learning

School psychologists have knowledge of individual differences, abilities, disabilities, and other diverse characteristics; principles and research related to diversity factors for children, families, and schools, including factors related to culture, context, and individual and role differences; and evidence-based strategies to enhance services and address potential influences related to diversity. School psychologists demonstrate skills to provide effective professional services that promote effective functioning for individuals, families, and schools with diverse characteristics, cultures, and backgrounds and across multiple contexts, with recognition that an understanding and respect for diversity in development and learning and advocacy for social justice are foundations for all aspects of service delivery.

Research and Program Evaluation

School psychologists have knowledge of research design, statistics, measurement, varied data collection and analysis techniques, and program evaluation sufficient for understanding research and interpreting data in applied settings. School psychologists demonstrate skills to evaluate and apply research as a foundation for service delivery and, in collaboration with others, use various techniques and technology resources for data collection, measurement, and analysis to support effective practices at the individual, group, and/or systems levels.

Continued

Table 1.2 (continued)   NASP Competency Domains (NASP, 2010)

Legal, Ethical, and Professional Practice
School psychologists have knowledge of the history and foundations of school psychology; multiple service models and methods; ethical, legal, and professional standards; and other factors related to professional identity and effective practice as school psychologists. School psychologists demonstrate skills to provide services consistent with ethical, legal, and professional standards; engage in responsive ethical and professional decision-making; collaborate with other professionals; and apply professional work characteristics needed for effective practice as school psychologists, including respect for human diversity and social justice, communication skills, effective interpersonal skills, responsibility, adaptability, initiative, dependability, and technology skills.

Source: Copyright 2010 by the National Association of School Psychologists, Bethesda, MD. Reprinted with permission of the publisher. www.nasponline.org

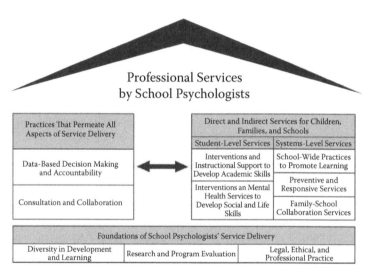

Figure 1.2   Model of comprehensive and integrated school psychological services. (Copyright 2010 by the National Association of School Psychologists, Bethesda, MD. Reprinted with permission of the publisher. www.nasponline.org)

Two

The Continuum
of Services Within
a Public Health Model

In our efforts to enhance children's academic outcomes, we have sometimes overlooked one of the basic prerequisites: attending to the mental health needs of children. Children who are stressed, distracted, or simply have not had the opportunity to learn self-care may have trouble getting along with others, feel unsafe in the classroom, or struggle to concentrate on their studies (de Voursney, Mannix, Brounstein, & Blau, 2008). Unfortunately, the resources available to meet these growing needs are limited because of a lack of mental health personnel such as school psychologists within the schools (Curtis, Chesno Grier, & Hunley, 2003). School personnel sometimes find themselves at a loss as to how to provide all of the different services that a student or family might need. Yet, it is also understood that to truly afford a child access to an education, it is imperative that the barriers to learning be removed. To accomplish the goals of academic and social–emotional success, a broad continuum of mental health support is a critical component of today's educational environments (Adelman & Taylor, 2009).

The challenge for our educational system is to find a framework of service that incorporates strategies for supporting healthy social–emotional development for all children, providing targeted, evidence-based services for children who need higher levels of support, and incorporating and aligning these services to be congruent with the context of schools and the goal of increased academic achievement. One such framework is provided by the Institute of Medicine (IOM). The IOM is the branch of the National Academy of Sciences that is responsible for health-related information and policy advice to governmental agencies and the public. Data and reports from the IOM are often used to guide public policy and public health initiatives. As noted in Chapter 1, both public health models and the NASP Practice Model support tiered levels of services to support individuals with different levels of needs. In 2009, the IOM introduced a continuum of mental health that outlines services from health promotion to management of chronic illness. Each of those components is discussed in the following sections with examples of school-based applications.

HEALTH PROMOTION

Early definitions of primary prevention focused on two elements: (1) preventing the occurrence of psychological problems, and (2) building psychological wellness (e.g., Cowen, 1973). The latter component is often referred to as *mental health promotion* and focuses exclusively on positive outcomes. Although it is recognized that programs that promote child wellness and healthy development might also prevent disorders, prevention is not the primary goal of health promotion. Positive youth development programs represent a good example of a mental health promotion approach (Catalano et al., 2004). Generally, the goals of these programs are to promote multiple competencies; foster self-determination, self-efficacy, and hope; and recognize positive and prosocial behaviors. As might be expected, positive youth development programs that were effective in building social, emotional, and cognitive competencies (e.g., self-determination, self-efficacy), were also effective in reducing drug and alcohol abuse, violence, and aggression (Catalano et al., 2004). That said, promoting health is valuable, regardless of whether someone also has mental illness or risk-taking behaviors. For instance, for a student with depression, development of self-expression through art or music is viewed as important from a health promotion perspective, independent of its impact on his or her affective issues.

Prevention, which places an emphasis on reducing or preventing a negative outcome, is relatively easier to study than promotion. Researchers could demonstrate that their programs reduced the incidence of specific disorders, but positive outcomes (e.g., higher levels of social–emotional competency) were more difficult to establish. Furthermore, funding sources

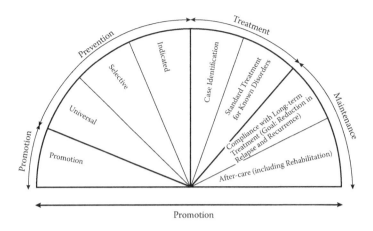

Figure 2.1   Public health model levels of services. (Reprinted from "Preventing mental, emotional, and behavioral disorders among young people: Progress and possibilities," by the National Research Council and Institute of Medicine, 2009, p. 67. Copyright 2009 by the National Research Council and Institute of Medicine. Reprinted with permission.)

were able to see the benefit of reducing the incidence of a disorder more so than the benefit of promoting a defined positive outcome. As a result, despite early recognition of the importance of promotion, the intervening years reflected a greater emphasis on prevention. More recently, prevention researchers have again argued for a combination of both prevention and promotion approaches to enhance mental health outcomes for youth (e.g., Cowen, 2000; Durlak & Wells, 1997; Greenberg et al., 2003). With the newest report, *Preventing Mental, Emotional, and Behavioral Disorders Among Young People*, the National Research Council (NRC) and IOM (2009) shifted their perspective by noting that "mental health promotion can be distinguished from prevention of mental disorders by its focus on healthy outcomes, such as competence and well-being, and that many of these outcomes are intrinsically valued in their own right" (p. 65). In fact, the new conceptualization of the mental health prevention spectrum begins with an emphasis on health promotion as illustrated in Figure 2.1.

With this new focus, emphasis is placed on the promotion of mental, emotional, and behavioral health as well as the prevention of mental health disorders. Program developers are encouraged to include both components, as it is believed that this type of dual emphasis leads to more effective programming (Greenberg et al., 2003). Furthermore, participating in health promotion activities may be less stigmatizing for children and their families, thus leading to increased levels of participation (NRC & IOM, 2009).

PREVENTION SCIENCE

Over the past 20 years, the field of prevention science has experienced tremendous growth. Prevention science refers to the rigorous study of the factors that are associated with negative outcomes. For example, it is well established that individuals who have been abused as children are more likely than those who did not experience abuse to have significant negative outcomes (e.g., substance abuse, more unstable relationships, depression; MacMillan et al., 2001). From a prevention perspective, rather than placing all of our service efforts into treating individuals who have experienced abuse, an alternative is to reduce the incidence of child abuse. The relationship between various risk factors and outcomes is extremely complex, and it has only been through careful study that we have developed greater knowledge of risk and resiliency as related to psychological, social, physical, and environmental factors (NRC & IOM, 2009; Weissberg, Kumpfer, & Seligman, 2003). (In Chapter 6 we provide a more complete presentation of various risk and protective factors).

The goal of prevention science is to develop a clear understanding of the pathway from risk factor to outcome, including the various intervening variables that act as catalysts or buffers, and then to use this information as the foundation for intervention programming and policy development (Doll & Yoon, 2010). In fact, research tells us that many interventions exist that can promote children's positive development and prevent emotional and behavioral problems (Kellam & Langevin, 2003; Pumariega & Winters, 2003; Weisz, Sandler, Durlak, & Anton, 2005). In their review of several prevention programs, Weisz et al. (2005) found that children who participated in these programs continued to demonstrate positive behaviors years later.

Many of these empirically supported programs may already be familiar to those working in schools. Programs such as Second Step (Committee for Children, 2010), Promoting Alternative Thinking Strategies [PATHS]; Kusché & Greenberg, 1994), and School-Wide Positive Behavioral Supports [now referred to as School-Wide Positive Behavioral Interventions and Supports, or simply PBIS] (Horner, Sugai, Todd, &

Lewis-Palmer, 2005) are all designed to address the needs of an entire school and to prevent negative outcomes (e.g., bullying, poor problem-solving, disruptive behavior). In addition to reducing the likelihood of emotional and behavioral problems, many of these programs have also been shown to be cost-effective because they result in decreased school absences, fewer special education placements, and reduced levels of incarceration or out-of-home placements (Aos, Lieb, Mayfield, Miller, & Punnuci, 2004).

Unfortunately, not all districts have adopted these types of programs; instead, they continue to rely on fragmented programs and materials, or to grab on to the newest program. Relatively little training is provided to district leaders, principals, teachers, and other service providers on how to select the most appropriate, empirically supported prevention programming that will effectively serve the needs of a specific population. A second barrier to implementing evidence-based prevention programming is that it has been difficult to create a shift in perspective from focusing on the needs of one child to serving a broader group of students. Yet, in order to address the mental health needs of children in the school, it is just this "shift" that is required. As George Albee (1989) aptly noted, "No mass disorder afflicting humankind has ever been eliminated or brought under control by attempts at treating the affected individual" (p. 373).

The original spectrum of mental health, developed in 1994 by the IOM, provided a common language for addressing prevention, treatment, and maintenance efforts in the field of mental health. This spectrum also featured prevention provided at three levels: universal, selective, and indicated (IOM, 1994). In making a decision whether to provide an intervention, the system (e.g., school district, community health department) must consider the risk of developing a particular problem weighed against the cost, risk, and inconvenience of the preventive intervention (IOM, 1994). For example, before deciding on whether to provide a time-intensive program to reduce bullying or increase problem-solving behavior, a needs analysis must first determine whether it is likely that these issues are a concern in a particular school or district. To what degree are students in the school experiencing bullying behaviors? What is the prevalence of certain kinds of problems (e.g., substance abuse, truancy) that might suggest that students are not engaging in good decision-making and/or problem-solving?

In addition to prevalence, the timing and cost of services must be considered. The IOM incorporated the work of R. Gordon (1987), who proposed a classification system based on levels of symptom severity and a corresponding cost-benefit formula. According to this system, the earliest levels of prevention (i.e., universal), require the least amount of cost per person and can be delivered by individuals who have only general expertise. From a school perspective, this means that paraprofessionals, teachers, and parents can all be active in delivering prevention efforts. As one moves up the prevention continuum and the level of risk for a particular population grows, the relative cost of intervention increases, as does the expertise needed from those delivering the intervention.

Levels of Prevention

This continuum of services is based on a system of levels that are designed to meet specific needs of the population. Many of the more familiar educational models, such as Response to Intervention [RtI] (Burns & Gibbons, 2008) and SWPBS [PBIS] (Horner et al., 2005), have adopted aspects of a public health model by creating tiered levels of prevention and intervention. It is important to keep in mind that we have presented only one of the tiered models; others exist that are helpful in conceptualizing levels of prevention (such as primary prevention, risk reduction, early intervention, and treatment; Meyers, 2002). It is also important to keep in mind that there is overlap in the boundaries between programs designed for the different levels (i.e., universal, selective). That is, there are often elements of the program that can be adapted in delivery intensity and focus to address groups who need greater levels of support. To better understand these different levels of prevention (i.e., universal, selective, indicated), a review of each, with relevant examples, is provided below.

Universal prevention. At a universal prevention level, no children are identified as having special needs or problems; instead, a positive foundation is created that supports the greatest number of children. In other words, all students are provided with the supports or programming through school- or district-wide practices and reform. For example, within a school setting, primary prevention would be directed toward creating school environments that support student learning and decrease children's risk for learning and/or behavioral problems. Adelman and Taylor (2000) have labeled this approach in the school setting as an *enabling component*. They describe this component as a comprehensive, multifaceted approach for addressing barriers to learning by providing a range of activities that promote healthy development for all students.

From this perspective, programs are designed to broadly address the underlying causal factors that are associated with negative outcomes. For example, schools that have high levels of bullying, where verbal harassment is tolerated, and where rules are perceived to be unfairly administered experience higher rates of truancy and school dropout (Ma, Phelps, Lerner, & Lerner, 2009). Rather than attempting to identify those students who are missing the most days of school and providing an intervention, a universal approach would address the broad needs of the system and the students. In response to this situation, the building leadership team might implement a problem-solving curriculum into health classes, reevaluate and align discipline practices, and train faculty to consistently address verbal threats and harassment. Through these low-cost and low-effort actions, it is expected that all students would experience a more positive school climate. To evaluate the effectiveness, data related to truancy rates, disciplinary actions, and school climate surveys could be collected to determine whether the changes are having the desired impact.

One of the more familiar universal educational programs is SWPBS [PBIS] (Horner et al., 2005). Although a full application of the program addresses all levels (i.e., universal through indicated), implementation of the universal level is most widespread. At this level, school personnel work together to establish common behavioral expectations across all school settings, students are taught the skills needed to meet these expectations, and students are consistently encouraged to and reinforced for engaging in the appropriate behavior. Building leadership teams use office referrals, attendance, and other sources of data to determine whether the program is having the desired effect (i.e., improving student behavior). Sugai and Horner (2008) estimated that when a school has a safe, supportive environment in which social and behavioral expectations are clearly communicated and consistently followed, 80% to 90% of children will respond favorably and need no additional supports. When schools engage in the development and implementation of positive school-wide behavioral interventions and supports, they are able to reduce behavioral referrals, increase academic achievement, and increase the degree to which school personnel work together (Bradshaw,

Koth, Bevans, Ialongo, & Leaf, 2008; Horner et al., 2005; Lassen, Steele, & Sailor, 2006).

All policy or program changes should be research based and the outcomes monitored regularly. In turn, these data are used to guide ongoing professional development and decision-making. As can be seen in the example above, rather than viewing one or more students as the target of intervention, the goal of primary or universal prevention is to enhance the environment so that it promotes the learning and well-being of all students. As noted by Rutter and Maughan (2002), "pupil achievement and behavior can be influenced (for better or worse) by the overall characteristics of the school environment" (p. 470).

Implementation of any school-wide approach also requires collaborative team planning in which a group of individuals (e.g., parents, teachers, administrators) come together to review the data, analyze, describe, and prioritize the problems, and create specific, measurable outcomes for their schools. Then, the team selects various evidence-based approaches to meet these goals. In effect, a problem-solving process is followed by the team to make decisions about systemic prevention efforts. Table 2.1 provides a few examples of evidence-based prevention programs designed to be provided at the universal level. These approaches are preventive and address the needs of the broadest range of children.

Selective prevention. Despite our best efforts at creating environments that support the needs of all students, there will

Table 2.1 Examples of Universal Programming

Universal Level of Prevention[a]	
Sample Programs	**Program Goals**
School-Wide Positive Behavioral Interventions and Supports (Horner et al., 2005)	Teach and consistently promote the use of appropriate social behaviors and reduce occurrence of problem behaviors.
Second Step (Committee for Children, 2010)	Teach students social-emotional competencies related to empathy, social problem-solving, and anger management.
Positive Alternatives for Thinking Strategies (PATHS; Kusché & Greenberg, 1994)	Reinforce and strengthen the use of self-regulation, self-determination, and problem-solving skills.
Social Decision Making/Social Problem Solving (Elias, Bruene-Butler, Bruno, Papke, & Shapiro, 2005)	Increase competency among elementary-age students by helping them to use their emotions to solve problems across various settings.

[a] This list is not meant to be all-inclusive, only to provide examples of universal programs.

be some children who require greater levels of mental health support because of internal and external factors that place them at greater risk for one or more negative outcomes. At the most basic level, gender, age, and socioeconomic status might place a child at risk. For example, females entering middle school frequently experience a reduction in their self-esteem, and children who enter school from households with limited incomes are often at risk for falling behind academically. Rather than addressing the needs of each student through individualized programming, selective prevention would be provided to the subgroup that has some common risk factor that increases their vulnerability to negative outcomes. With selective prevention, also referred to as targeted prevention, the screening efforts required to identify groups that might be "at risk" can be minimal. The Head Start preschool program is an excellent example of a selective prevention. Students and their families qualify for this program based on income; there is no need to establish that the child is struggling behaviorally or academically. Because many preschool children from low-income families are at risk for poor educational and health outcomes (Ramey & Ramey, 1998), this program was designed to help families support their child's healthy development (Zigler & Muenchow, 1992).

Interventions targeted at this level are sometimes considered to be a form of early intervention because a potential problem is identified and additional supports are provided. However, at this level, students only demonstrate risk or vulnerability rather than a full clinical manifestation of a disorder. The program is delivered to address the needs of the subgroup as a whole, rather than targeting specific students. Because not all students will receive the intervention, this approach is considered to be selective rather than universal. These types of programs are also typically low cost to school districts because of the limited amount of screening necessary and lower level of intervention intensity, either in duration or frequency. Program goals at this level of prevention are focused on reducing or eliminating the onset of problems or negative outcomes by addressing causal factors *for the group.*

Several effective targeted prevention programs have been identified for use in school and community settings. For example, antisocial behaviors have been effectively addressed through programs that focus on improving skills in problem-solving, decision-making, peer resistance, stress management, and academic performance (Botvin & Kantor, 2000; Stephens,

1998). Skill-building programs typically include a series of structured lessons that incorporate role plays, adult and peer modeling, and applied practice in real-life contexts (e.g., Greenberg & Kusché, 2006; Shure & Spivack, 1988).

Another example of an effective selective intervention is the Talking with TJ program, based on the Social Decision Making/Social Problem Solving program (Elias, Bruene-Butler, Bruno, Papke, & Shapiro, 2005; Elias, Gara, Ubriaco, & Rothbaum, 1986; Rosenblatt & Elias, 2008). All students who are about to transition to middle school would qualify for the selected subgroup. This program was designed to ease the transition from elementary to middle school. Practitioners and researchers alike have long recognized the difficulties that students face with the transition from the elementary to the secondary level, including a drop in grade point average (GPA), social isolation, and increased behavioral challenges (Alspaugh, 1998; Seidman, Allen, Aber, & Mitchell, 1994). The goal of this program is to reduce the drop in academic achievement that is often seen as students move to a middle school setting. In one study, Talking to TJ was delivered to 145 fifth-grade students who received this social-emotional curriculum for a year prior to transitioning to sixth grade (Rosenblatt & Elias, 2008). It was found that when the program ended, all students had experienced a drop in their GPAs. However, those who had received the greatest exposure to the program experienced a smaller decrease in their GPAs than those who had received the least exposure. Similar transition programs have been shown to reduce social problems among young adolescents transitioning to middle school (e.g., Coping Power Program; Lochman & Wells, 2002).

There are also situations in which children must adjust to significant changes in their families (e.g., divorce, job loss, incarceration), which can create increased levels of risk. Support programs such as divorce groups, coping skills training, and other forms of support can help children adjust to these new life circumstances. Selected interventions can be provided through group approaches with the focus on change within the students who participate in the group (e.g., increased coping), or can be focused on the context by enhancing the supports around the student. For example, the Children of Divorce Intervention Program [CODIP] (Pedro-Carroll & Cowen, 1987) was designed to help youth experiencing family divorce to obtain support from their peers and learn coping skills. The program has been modified and adapted to address the needs of children from Kindergarten through Grade 8. Research across various age groups has supported its effectiveness in increasing school engagement and decreasing problem behaviors at home and school (Alpert-Gillis, Pedro-Carroll, & Cowen, 1989; Pedro-Carroll & Alpert-Gillis, 1997; Pedro-Carroll, Cowen, Hightower, & Guare, 1986).

Selective prevention can address subgroups of students directly or can address the surrounding system, such as the family, school, or peer group. Parent education programs that help families to become more involved in their child's education or develop more consistent discipline at home are examples of selective prevention programs that focus on contexts rather than individuals. Table 2.2 provides a sample of Tier 2 mental health programs that have been successfully implemented in school settings.

Fortunately, a separate program is not necessarily required for each type of risk. If you examine the theories that underlie the programs, many address similar core components and help individuals to develop a broad range of skills. Therefore, one type of program might be used to address seemingly different groups of youth (e.g., those with depressive symptoms and those at risk for substance abuse). Additionally, programs might be integrated to address a greater level of need. One example of this integrated model was provided by Domitrovich et al. (2010), who blended a refined version of the Good Behavior Game (Embry, Staatemeier, Richardson, Lauger, & Mitich, 2003) with PATHS (Kusché & Greenberg, 1994) to address the needs of students in

Table 2.2   Examples of Selective Programs

Selective Level of Prevention[a]	
Sample Programs	**Program Goals**
Coping Power Program (Lochman, Wells, & Lenhart, 2008)	Teach students (early adolescents) to recognize their feelings and deal with them appropriately without displaying aggressive behaviors.
Talking with TJ (Rosenblatt & Elias, 2008)	Reduce the drop in academic achievement as students transition from elementary to middle school.
Children of Divorce Intervention Program (CODIP; Pedro-Carroll & Cowen, 1987)	Increase coping skills and group support for children (Grades K–5) who have experienced divorce in their families.
Strengthening Families Program: For Parents and Youth 10–14 (Molgaard & Spoth, 2001)	Improve youth and parent competencies, increase parenting skills, and reduce substance use in young adolescents.

[a]   This list is not meant to be all-inclusive, only to provide examples of selective programs.

high-risk, urban schools. By integrating prevention programs, schools are able to provide high-quality programming in a more efficient manner with greater levels of fidelity and possibly receive additional benefits (Domitrovich et al., 2010). An initial pilot study supported high levels of satisfaction and perceived positive changes in student behavior with the integrated program; an ongoing randomized control trial is under way.

Indicated prevention. Further along the public health continuum, focus is directed toward those individuals who are demonstrating early manifestations of challenging behaviors, difficulty managing their emotions, and social isolation. These behaviors might be viewed as early indicators of long-term disorders that, if not treated early, will go on to develop into disabling conditions. Therefore, programs designed for the indicated level of prevention tend to be more comprehensive and to target many different aspects of the individual's environment. Additionally, most of the prevention programming is delivered to small groups but will also typically have an individual component built in. Because students have not responded to previous prevention programming and have greater severity in their behavioral or emotional symptoms, a great amount of time, effort, and resources is required to provide prevention programming at this level. Despite this cost in terms of time, energy, and programming, these types of programs are considered to be cost effective in the long term (NRC & IOM, 2009).

Children with early-onset behavioral problems are at greater risk for antisocial behaviors, poor academic achievement, school dropout, and substance abuse (Costello, Foley, & Angold, 2006; Egger & Angold, 2006). Aggression in particular appears to be a long-standing problem and, if not addressed by Grade 3, is likely to persist into adulthood and result in negative outcomes (Crick et al., 2006). In fact, Petras et al. (2008) concluded that if you want to reduce adolescent risk behaviors, the single generic risk factor that is best to target in elementary school is aggression. Thus, if we intervene earlier, we reduce the likelihood that patterns of aggression, substance abuse, and social isolation will become a chronic challenge for this relatively small number of students who do not respond to universal prevention programming.

Prevention for those behaviors that pose significant risk to individuals can be implemented at any age, but the majority of evidence-based programs focus on preschool and elementary-age populations (e.g., Incredible Years, Webster-Stratton, 1982;

Fast Track, Conduct Problems Prevention Research Group, 1999). The Incredible Years program was originally designed for children ages 3 to 8. Over the years, it has grown into a comprehensive package that includes teacher training in effective classroom management, parent training in creating a positive home environment, and a curriculum of 60 lessons designed to enhance the social–emotional development of children (Webster-Stratton & Herman, 2010). This program has been demonstrated to be effective in reducing levels of aggressive behavior in young children. In fact, it is one of 11 programs recognized by the Office for Juvenile Justice and Delinquency Prevention (OJJDP) as an evidence-based intervention for preventing and treating disruptive behavior.

The Fast Track project (Conduct Problems Prevention Research Group, 1999) also represents a comprehensive prevention program that was designed to reduce disruptive behaviors in children who are at the highest risk of developing conduct disorders. The project provides an excellent example of a comprehensive, public health approach. After screening approximately 10,000 children, 891 were identified as being at high risk for conduct disorder. The program provides components for the home, school, and child that are directed toward reducing risk and enhancing protective factors. Some of the program elements delivered in early adolescence include tutoring, mentoring, home visits, and involvement in community programs. Recent evaluations of the program have found decreases in aggression, lower levels of harsh parenting practices, and positive gains in social, cognitive, and academic skills (Nix, Pinderhughes, Bierman, Maples, and the Conduct Problems Prevention Research Group, 2005).

Although the previous two examples feature comprehensive programming that targets multiple contexts in the child's life, some programs are narrower in scope and focus on helping youth to develop skills related to a targeted area. In their meta-analysis of prevention efforts for reducing depressive symptoms, Horowitz and Garber (2006) reported that selective and indicated programs were more effective than universal programs at reducing depressive symptoms in youth. In fact, Cuijpers, van Straten, Smit, Mihalopoulos, and Beekman (2008) found that preventive interventions for adolescents reduced the incidence of depressive disorders by 23%. These two studies included a variety of approaches that were mostly based on cognitive–behavioral interventions. An example of such a program is the Clarke Cognitive–Behavioral Prevention

Intervention, which targets adolescents who are at risk for developing major depression. The program has demonstrated promising results in several randomized trials (Clarke et al., 1995, 2001). It is designed to be delivered over 15 sessions in a small group format in a school setting. It is modeled after other cognitive–behavioral interventions to treat depression and focuses on helping adolescents to cope with stress.

Additional services such as individual and group counseling, functional–behavioral assessment, and ongoing consultation may be needed for those children who are at the "indicated" level of prevention. In addition to contextual interventions such as positive school-wide behavioral supports and skill training through group interventions, these children and their families often require expanded services through community agencies. Intensive, focused services through school/community networks are necessary for the small percentage of children and their families who are experiencing significant challenges (Sugai & Horner, 2008). Table 2.3 details a few evidence-based programs designed to be delivered in school settings at the indicated level of intervention.

Efficacy of Primary Prevention

There is ample evidence to suggest that prevention works. Not only are there hundreds of studies that evaluate the outcomes of specific prevention programs, but there are also a number of meta-analyses and systematic reviews that demonstrate the

Table 2.3 Examples of Indicated Programs

Indicated Level of Prevention[a]	
Sample Programs	Program Goals
Incredible Years (Webster-Stratton, 1982)	Reduce disruptive behaviors and improve social–emotional competence in preschool children by increasing classroom management skills in teachers, behavior management strategies in parents, and providing a curriculum delivered in a small group or whole classroom environment.
Clarke Cognitive–Behavioral Prevention Intervention (Clarke et al., 1995)	Increase coping skills in adolescents at risk for developing major depression through use of cognitive–behavioral approaches.
Fast Track (Conduct Problems Prevention Research Group, 1999)	Reduce risk factors and promote skill development in children who are at risk for conduct disorders and their families.

[a] This list is not meant to be all-inclusive, only to provide examples of indicated programs.

effectiveness of prevention programming (NRC & IOM, 2009). For example, Durlak and Wells (1997) conducted a comprehensive meta-analysis of 177 primary prevention programs with children and adolescents. They concluded that programs that modified the school environment, helped students manage stressful transitions, and provided individualized mental health promotion resulted in significant, positive changes in student competencies and reduced problem behaviors. In fact, there is evidence for the efficacy of primary prevention in the areas of behavioral and social problems, learning problems, alcohol and drug abuse, physical health problems, injuries, and child abuse (Durlak, 1995, 1997; Greenberg et al., 2003).

Furthermore, prevention efforts directed at systemic change (e.g., school and classroom environment, parenting practices) also resulted in positive outcomes. In a meta-analysis of universal-level competence-promotion studies, Durlak et al. (2007) reported that many of the programs that attempted to create systemic change were able to demonstrate significant changes. However, follow-up data were not available in many of the studies so it was difficult to determine whether these positive outcomes were maintained. One notable exception was in the area of parenting practices. Follow-up data from 17 studies suggested that parenting practices continued to be significantly stronger (effect size = .49) after prevention efforts. Although there are effective school-based prevention programs available at all levels of the IOM model, much of the research has focused on universal programs implemented during the early elementary school years and have measured individual rather than systemic outcomes (Durlak et al., 2007).

INTENSIVE SERVICES IN CHILDREN'S MENTAL HEALTH

Despite our best efforts to build and maintain effective health promotion and prevention programs, some students will develop mental health problems. One of the most recent estimates of mental health disorders in children reported a prevalence rate of 17% (with ranges from 12% to 22%) of mental, emotional, or behavioral disorders among youth (NRC & IOM, 2009). In other words, in an average large high school of 2,000 students, it would be expected that 340 of these adolescents would be struggling with some type of mental health problem severe enough to cause distress. Many of these students will likely have first experienced their symptoms in elementary or middle school. In a national survey of adults, nearly half of adults affected by mental health problems reported symptoms of serious mental illness prior to age 14 (Kessler et al., 2005).

The most common disorders affecting children and adolescents include disruptive behavior disorders, substance abuse and dependence, depressive disorders, and anxiety disorders (Costello, Mustillo, Keller, & Angold, 2004). The Surgeon General's Report (U.S. Department of Health and Human Services, 1999) predicted that the rate of mental health problems in children would increase by 50% during the next 20 years in part due to the lack of appropriate preventive mechanisms, faulty early identification procedures (which precludes appropriate early intervention), and fragmented service delivery. Despite these various estimates, the actual prevalence of child and adolescent psychiatric disorders is unknown. Instead, these figures represent estimates based on smaller studies (50 surveys from around the world from 1992 to 2002) using different methods and time frames (Costello et al., 2004).

Within the school setting, students with emotional difficulties, which often reflect clinical disorders, are identified as having Serious Emotional Disturbance (SED). Students with SED may or may not be formally diagnosed but are recognized as having emotional and/or behavioral difficulties that negatively impact their ability to function in an educational setting. Historically, these youth have not fared well in school. Compared to students with other disabilities, students with SED have higher rates of school dropout and academic failure. Furthermore, they are more likely to become involved in the juvenile justice system, to be poor, to be unemployed, to abuse substances, and to have a child during their adolescent years (Bullis & Cheney, 1999; Carson, Sitlington, & Frank, 1995; Kern, Hilt-Panahon, & Sokol, 2009; U.S. Department of Education, 2005).

The range of students identified as such varies greatly. In their review of seven data sets, Costello et al. (1998) found that between 4% and 7% of children in the United States had SED. An earlier review by Friedman et al. (1996) estimated the range to be closer to 9% to 12%. In their most recent work, Costello et al. (2004) reported the current median estimate to be 11.3%. Unfortunately, of the students identified with SED, only 1 in 4 received any type of professional mental health care during their most recent episode (i.e., acute expression of symptoms), and only half had ever received any services (Costello et al., 1996, 1998; Kataoka, Zhang, & Wells, 2002).

Whereas many of these disorders may be mild and of a relatively short duration, the more serious disorders tend to be long-lasting and have a negative effect on overall functioning (Friedman et al., 1996; Kessler, Foster, Saunders, & Stang, 1995). One additional factor that complicates services to children and adolescents is that of *comorbidity*, or the occurrence of more than one disorder. One of the central characteristics of psychiatric disorders of children and adolescents is the high level of comorbidity (Costello et al., 2004), which suggests that, for children, being at risk for one disorder places them at risk for others. The highest levels of comorbidity were among children served in the school setting (Garland et al., 2001). As might be expected, children with comorbid disorders are more likely to have greater levels of functional impairment. Therefore, a model of service that incorporates a broad range of services consistent with the IOM spectrum is needed within the school setting.

Treatment for Students in a Public Health Model

Just as there is a continuum of prevention, once a child has been identified as having a mental illness, there continues to be a range of services needed that can effectively treat and enhance that individual's level of functioning. According to the IOM spectrum of mental health, services at the treatment level of intervention include case identification and standard treatment for disorders. At the maintenance level, issues of stabilizing functioning, rehabilitation, and aftercare are addressed. In many ways, these levels of service mirror the traditional practice of school psychologists, in that their efforts have often been directed toward identifying students with special learning and emotional needs and then assisting those students as they progress through their education. At these more intensive levels, school psychologists' work is directed toward the individual child and the system (e.g., family, classroom teacher, peers) around that child.

Case Identification

Current practices tend to favor waiting until a child's behavior is considerably outside the norm before providing identification or diagnosis for fear of mislabeling a child. Unfortunately, because services are often tied to diagnosis, early intervention programming is limited. There is also tension between school and community service providers over the issue of identification strategies. In the community, the *Diagnostic and Statistical Manual of Mental Disorders* (*DSM-IV*) provides the codes and language for identification, and community practitioners use this reference to diagnose children in order to receive reimbursement for their services. Within the schools, not only is there a different method for identifying SED, but there is also a disincentive for doing so because of the relatively higher educational cost of children with special needs. In fact, Friedman et al. (2004) suggested that only about 1% of children nationally (about 500,000 per year) are identified as having SED, a figure that is much lower than expected, given national prevalence rates. There appears to be a significant underidentification of mental health needs in the schools.

Returning to our typical high school with approximately 340 students who are struggling with mild to severe symptoms of depression, anxiety, substance abuse, eating disorders, behavioral difficulties, or some combination of these, we would find about 30 to 37 students would qualify for specialized services for their emotional disability. Based on the findings from earlier studies, about 85 (~25%) would receive some sort of support through available school and community services (e.g., counseling at the school, peer mentoring, community mental health providers, private providers). Using these estimates, that means that over 200 students would continue to struggle with their symptoms without benefit of mental health services. This discrepancy in identification and treatment practices begins with the lack of a systematic identification method and results in the unmet needs of too many students in our schools.

Universal screening is one strategy that can be used to identify students who might benefit from early intervention strategies (Levine, Perkins, & Perkins, 2005). Historically, schools have not been willing to implement widespread screening of social–emotional or behavioral functioning. Too often, nonacademic problems were given lower priority and not viewed as the responsibility of the school. For example, Lloyd, Kaufman, Landrum, and Roe (1991) found that the peak referral period for academic problems occurred in second or third grade, whereas the peak referral time for behavioral concerns occurred in ninth grade (Walker, Nishioka, Zeller, Severson, & Feil, 2000). With the advent of tiered intervention models such as Positive Behavioral Interventions and Supports, and Response to Intervention, there has been an increasing openness to the idea of universal screening for emotional and behavioral concerns (Severson, Walker, Hope-Doolittle, Kratochwill, & Gresham, 2007).

There are also opponents to school-based screening who raise concerns over the potential stigmatization of students (Levitt, Saka, Romanelli, & Hoagwood, 2007); the validity of the instruments (Barbarin, 2007); and parental concerns about labeling, consent, and schools exceeding their boundaries. Instead, most children with emotional or behavioral problems come to the attention of their family physician. In fact, one of the best indicators of risk for developing a mental health disorder is a concern about a child's behavior on the part of the parent or guardian (NRC & IOM, 2009). Therefore, one of the simplest screening methods that physicians (or school personnel) might use is to ask parents about their concerns. Unfortunately, many physicians are not well trained in screening for mental health or behavioral issues, are not linked to community behavioral health resources, and are not typically reimbursed for behavioral screening (NRC & IOM, 2009). With the current system, we have limited mechanisms for identifying students who are at risk or showing early manifestations of a disorder and who would benefit from preventive or early intervention approaches.

To implement a public health model, we must work to develop a reliable and valid method of case identification within the school system. One program that has received empirical support is the Systematic Screening for Behavior Disorders (SSBD; Walker & Severson, 1990). Students are screened through a number of "gates" involving teacher nominations, ratings, and direct observations. Those students who at the highest levels (i.e., top three) of each of these lists are typically referred for selective or indicated level of prevention. Preliminary evidence suggested that this instrument was able to reliably differentiate those students with behavior disorders from those without (Elliott & Busse, 2004). Another screening instrument, the Social Skills Improvement System: Rating Scales (SSIS-RS; Gresham & Elliott, 2008), focuses on social behaviors, since social deficits are associated with numerous disorders. The SSIS-RS also provides a tiered model of social skills interventions that can be provided to those students who are struggling with social skill performance or acquisition deficits by building on their strengths (Gresham & Elliott, 2008; Gresham, Elliott, Vance, & Cook, 2011).

Identifying students who are at the subthreshold (indicated level) of need may be one strategy for accurately identifying those students who are most at risk for developing mental, emotional, and/or behavioral disorders. A 15-year longitudinal study by Shankman et al. (2009) revealed that those individuals who were at the subthreshold for many conditions (e.g., anxiety, depression, substance abuse and conduct) went on to develop the full syndrome. Thus targeting students who are at the subthreshold of qualifying for a disorder may allow for indicated prevention/early intervention for those individuals who are most at risk. Using this method, Walker et al. (2009) identified students in an urban district who were rated among their teachers as most aggressive. The researchers completed a randomized, control trial and reported that after receiving an intervention that focused on parenting skills and classroom interventions, those identified students significantly improved in symptoms, function, and academic outcomes.

Standard Treatment for Disorders
After a student is identified as qualifying for special services, the most effective interventions will be time intensive and are sometimes beyond the scope of the school system alone. By having an established network of community connections, school-based providers can link students and families with community services that could better meet their needs. Community-based treatment can be costly in terms of both money and time. A public health model does not negate the need for this type of intervention when warranted. Instead, the focus is directed toward reducing the number of cases that require this level of resource utilization.

Despite this recognition that children with moderate to severe mental health needs are best served through intensive supports, schools remain one of the main providers of mental health services because many families lack access to community resources. Slade (2002) found that 4.4% of adolescents received mental health counseling in the school during a 1-year period, while 8.8% received service outside of the schools. Overall, school-based mental health interventions appear to be effective. Of the four published meta-analyses that have focused on school-based mental health services (Baskin et al., 2010; Prout & DeMartino, 1986; Prout & Prout, 1998; Reese, Prout, Zirkelback, & Anderson, 2010), all have reported medium to large effect sizes. One of the most recent studies was based on a review of 107 outcome studies of 132 interventions. Baskin et al. (2010) concluded that psychotherapy with children and adolescents in the schools yielded positive effects. Certain variables appeared to increase the effectiveness of counseling, including services provided to adolescent populations, single-gender groups, and trained, licensed therapists rather than paraprofessionals or graduate students providing the counseling (Baskin et al., 2010). Further, the modality did not appear to make a difference, as individual, group, and "other" approaches (e.g., classroom) all yielded significant results.

Another recent meta-analysis by Reese et al. (2010) reviewed 65 school-based psychotherapy and counseling dissertations and found similar results to those of Baskin et al. (2010). As with previous school-based studies, most of the interventions included those that focused on cognitive-behavioral strategies or skills training and were typically provided in a group format. These broad studies can help us to understand which aspects of counseling or psychotherapy have the strongest effects and the areas where we continue to have gaps in our knowledge. For example, whereas Prout and Prout (1998) and Reese et al. (2010) reported the largest effect sizes for elementary populations, Baskin et al. (2010) reported larger effect sizes for adolescents.

The inconsistent nature of these findings leads us to conclude that ongoing research on school-based interventions is needed to determine which approaches are most effective with whom. We also need to use a variety of methods to study these outcomes. For example, Weiss, Catron, Harris, and Phung (1999) used a randomized clinical trial to determine the effectiveness of child psychotherapy as typically delivered in the schools. Participants included 160 children who had problems related to anxiety, depression, aggression, or attention. They were divided into a treatment or control group that received either "treatment as usual" or academic tutoring for 45 minutes per week. Treatment as usual was provided by mental health professionals (six master's level counselors and one doctoral level clinical psychologist) who reported using cognitive and psychodynamic–humanistic approaches. The treatment extended over 2 years and did not follow a particular set of guidelines. At the end of the project, the researchers did not find any significant differences between the students in the two groups based on ratings of internalizing or externalizing behaviors, adaptive functioning, or peer relationships across time.

Within a school setting, it may not be possible to deliver evidence-based therapy or treatment with fidelity due to limitations in the setting. That is, it is difficult to pull students out of their coursework on a regular basis; there are often unexpected interruptions during the day (e.g., fire alarms, crises) that make it difficult to provide consistency; and it is sometimes simply not an appropriate setting (e.g., privacy limitations). Additionally, school mental health professionals (e.g., school psychologists, school social workers) may not be adequately prepared in the delivery of specific evidence-based treatment approaches. Some of these barriers may be addressed by delivering services after school through school-based clinics, or by creating partnerships between mental health professionals from local mental health centers who consult with the school.

Examples of school and community partnerships have been described in the literature on full-service schools, expanded school mental health, or school-based mental health services. In full-service schools and those with expanded school mental health services, a broad range of mental health services are offered to students and families through partnerships with community mental health agencies (Table 2.4 lists examples of these types of programs). The goals of these types of programs are to increase student attendance and achievement, as well as to enhance the overall quality of life for students through health (including mental health) programming and supports (Weist, Ambrose, & Lewis, 2006). These types of partnerships

Table 2.4 Examples of Collaborative Mental Health Programs for Youth

Mental Health Treatment Programs[a]	
Sample Programs	**Program Goals**
School Mental Health Program (Weist et al., 2006)	School program designed to increase student attendance and achievement and enhance overall quality of life
Partial Day Treatment (Robinson & Rapport, 2002)	Multimodal treatment designed to reduce behavioral symptoms while increasing self-management and problem-solving skills
Extended Day Treatment (Vanderploeg et al., 2009)	After school programming designed to assist students in building their social skills through milieu, individual, and family therapy
Multisystemic Therapy (Henggeler & Lee, 2003)	Intensive home-based but collaborative model designed to empower families and help families build skills and strengths

[a] This list is not meant to be all-inclusive, only to provide examples of collaborative mental health programs.

are beneficial to both parties: Schools are able to access additional personnel who can address the complex mental health needs of students, and community agencies are able to access a greater number of youth and their families (Weist et al., 2006). An example of this type of program exists through the School Mental Health Program operated through the University of Maryland, which provides services to 28 schools in Baltimore.

Another model that has been growing in popularity is day treatment programming that is offered by the school, often in partnership with a community mental health agency. For example, Robinson and Rapport (2002) reported on the effectiveness of a day treatment program delivered in a public school setting that provided mental health services to students. Many of the 142 participants had already been in resource, counseling, and inpatient settings. The multimodal treatment program was delivered through a community mental health program in collaboration with the school district. Intervention components were delivered through a multidisciplinary team that included a psychiatrist, psychologists, social workers, teachers, and behavioral aides. The programming was designed to reduce behavioral symptoms while increasing a variety of self-management and problem-solving skills by using behavioral techniques such as behavioral contracts, token economies based on a level system, and frequent feedback. Additional program components included weekly individual and family counseling sessions and medication management as needed. Academic instruction was delivered in classroom environments that were similar to others within the school in most ways except that the behavioral techniques were integrated into all aspects of the day treatment classrooms. Results of a year-long study indicated that 50.7% of the sample had reduced symptoms, and 25.7% scored below clinical cutoff levels, suggesting the effectiveness of this type of intensive, collaborative programming.

Alternatively, or in addition to, day treatment programming, Vanderploeg, Franks, Plant, Cloud, and Tebes (2009) have promoted the idea of Extended Day Treatment (EDT). In this model, students attend EDT as an after school program and students are able to receive individual and family therapy, as well as working with other youth in a milieu setting to build their social skills. This model is considered to be an intermediate level of center-based care that is indicated for youth who are at high risk of residential placement or who have not been successful in other types of programming.

Because it is offered after school, children and adolescents are able to remain in their homes, schools, and communities with minimal disruption. Although elements of this type of programming have evidence to support their use (e.g., day treatment, family involvement in therapy), there is not yet support for this type of programming overall. However, five states have adopted programs similar to EDT to help fill recognized service gaps (Vanderploeg et al., 2009).

A more systematically evaluated program for intervening with troubled youth in the community is Multisystemic Therapy (MST; Henggeler & Lee, 2003). This multimodal approach has focused primarily on juvenile offenders but has been applied effectively with youth with SED during a psychiatric crisis (Henggeler, Schoenwald, Rowland, & Cunningham, 2002). This empirically supported treatment is home based but relies on principles of collaboration of all systems in which the child is involved, empowerment of caregivers, and an intensity of services that are oriented to building skills and strengths in children and their families. This therapeutic model is intensive but also relatively short term (approximately 6 months). A substantial body of evidence suggests that MST is also effective in treating serious antisocial behavior in adolescents (U.S. Public Health Service, 2001).

The programs described in this section provide just a few examples of the types of programming that can be provided through partnership to meet the more intensive levels of children's mental health needs. School psychologists can play a key role in these partnerships by reaching out to local agencies, participating on interagency councils, and working with (or initiating) groups of stakeholders who have a common goal of addressing a problem area in the continuum of mental health services for children and youth in the community (described in more detail in Chapter 3). This continuum does not end with immediate treatment of the mental health crisis. For some youth, mental health issues may persist despite their having received appropriate treatment.

A form to assist in mapping current programs and resources is provided on the accompanying CD (2.1).

Maintenance in a Public Health Model

Chronic mental health problems may require an intensive, ongoing level of service. The original IOM model described three components that address the needs of individuals: stabilizing functioning, rehabilitation, and aftercare. More recently, Adelman and Taylor (2003) described the components to include referral, triage, placement guidance and assistance; case management and resource coordination; family preservation programs and services; special education and rehabilitation; dropout recovery and follow-up support; and/or services for severe-chronic psychosocial/mental/physical health problems. Children with the most severe needs are often served in multiple settings, including special education, social services, and juvenile justice (Friedman et al., 2004). Clearly, any one individual or system could not be expected to provide these services; instead, a comprehensive network is required to assist students, families, schools, and communities in addressing these identified problems.

Two promising approaches that have been promoted are a System of Care model (Stroul & Friedman, 1996) and, as a part of this model, the development of a Wraparound team process (Scott & Eber, 2003). A System of Care model emphasizes the development of a range of services, building partnerships between parents and service providers and between a variety of different community service agencies (e.g., social services, community mental health, juvenile justice). Through this model, children and families receive individualized, comprehensive, and culturally competent care that is designed at the local level using the best available research evidence (Stroul & Friedman, 1996). Culturally competent care that is designed at the local level is especially critical to meeting the mental health needs of children and families from diverse ethnic and linguistic backgrounds. According to the Surgeon General's supplemental report on mental health focusing on culture, race, and ethnicity (U.S. Department of Health and Human Services, 2001), individuals of color have less access to mental health services, are less likely to receive them, and receive poorer quality care as compared to Whites.

Wraparound represents a positive model of support for children and their families who are experiencing significant mental health needs and who are involved with different service systems (e.g., juvenile justice, social services, community mental health, school). All aspects of planning occur within a team identified by the family and caregivers, and the purpose is to develop a coordinated plan and support system across multiple systems (Eber, Sugai, Smith, & Scott, 2002; Stroul & Friedman, 1996). A recent meta-analysis, including seven studies evaluating the effectiveness of Wraparound services, indicated that those youth who were involved in Wraparound had better outcomes (small to medium effect size) than youth who received conventional services (Suter & Bruns, 2009).

School-based mental health professionals can be active participants in the Wraparound team and System of Care. Both of these approaches help to accomplish the goals of stabilizing an individual's functioning, providing for rehabilitation, and creating natural supports for long-term aftercare. With effective communication and expanded support networks, students with SED demonstrate improved outcomes across different educational settings (Eber & Nelson, 1997) and increased school completion (Malloy, Cheney, & Cormier, 1998). When a Wraparound process is used, families are able to build natural community supports to meet their needs. It is important to recognize that families may possess certain strengths and needs, but their ability to function effectively must also include the natural supports and resources in the environment. As Friedman et al. (2004) noted, "The challenge, therefore, in children's mental health is not just to develop treatments for the child, but to help develop the supports needed by the family and in the community to improve functioning and reduce impairment and stress" (p. 139). Furthermore, an interagency team model allows for more effective communication between all stakeholders around the needs of the child and family, and decreases the likelihood of duplication or significant service gaps (Eber et al., 2002).

PROMOTION, PREVENTION, AND TREATMENT IN A SOCIAL–ECOLOGICAL FRAMEWORK

Children are greatly affected by their environments. In designing mental health promotion, prevention, and intervention programs, we must consider the contexts that will impact the delivery as well as the effectiveness of these services. That is, none of these programs can exist in isolation from the social, family, political, and cultural systems that are a part of all communities (Keys & Leaf, 2008). When we consider risk, it is not the characteristics of the individual that place him or her at risk, but the interactions between the individual and the environment (E. W. Gordon, 2003). Therefore, Keys and Leaf noted that program development and evaluation need to be conducted at the level of society (e.g., policies, stigma), the organization (e.g., staff capacity), and the provider (e.g., fidelity of implementation). The causes of children's mental health problems are multiple and complex, but most often they include one or more of these factors: biological, psychological, and social.

A social–ecological model framework can serve as a template for a multi-level approach. In particular, Bronfenbrenner's (1979) ecological model can be used to conceptualize service delivery at different levels within a public health model. Because of all the complex links between the health of an individual and that of a system, it is recognized that an intervention directed solely at changing the individual is less likely to be successful than one that addresses the needs of the broader system (Weisz et al., 2005).

The ecological model considers four contextual environments that impact the individual: the microsystem, mesosystem, exosystem, and macrosystem (Bronfenbrenner, 1979). Although some interventions might be directed toward the individual, as noted above, that level of impact would not be considered sufficient or likely to be effective. The *microsystem* includes environments in which the child interacts on a daily basis, such as the home and classroom. The relationships between contexts (e.g., the parent's *interactions* with the school) are addressed in the *mesosystem*. The *exosystem* might be comprised of the family's socioeconomic status, the neighborhood, and the larger school system. Finally, the *macrosystem* includes the larger institutions and culture that directly or indirectly impact the individual, such as legislation, government programs, and the entire educational system. From this perspective, preventing mental health problems in youth is conceptualized as an ongoing mutual accommodation between the individual and the environment in which development occurs in the context of several interrelated systems (Bronfenbrenner, 1979).

In our conceptualization of a continuum of care, one end of the continuum would feature evidence-based promotion and prevention services that create a positive educational climate focused on learning. We can be confident that "well-designed, well-implemented school-based prevention and youth development programming can positively influence a diverse array of social, health and academic outcomes" (Greenberg et al., 2003, p. 470). These programs would address at least three levels of need and be delivered within a positive system of care framework that involves all stakeholders. It is recognized that this type of prevention programming cannot meet the needs of all students, especially those with an identified disorder.

However, this shift in thinking can go a long way in preventing future problems and in creating a positive foundation and supports for those students who are struggling with more serious disorders.

CONCLUSION

This brief review supports the need for an intensified focus on early intervention. By identifying risk and protective factors and incorporating this knowledge into our prevention efforts, we can possibly begin to reduce the incidence of mental health symptoms and disorders in child and adolescent populations. We are never going to eliminate mental health disorders but if we enhance levels of adaptation in children and youth, the need for greater levels of service will be greatly reduced. We propose that school-based practitioners create a *continuum of care* that reflects the IOM spectrum in order to increase the number of evidence-based services that students receive. Ideally, this continuum is woven into the fabric of the school to promote positive school environments, expand family and community partnerships, implement prevention programming, and partner with community agencies on treatment and follow-up care programming.

We can build this capacity through collaborative relationships with families and community agencies and interdisciplinary professional development opportunities. Intensive levels of social, emotional, behavioral, and academic needs are most effectively addressed when school-based service providers, families, and representatives of other mental health professions work together. Unfortunately, our current approaches do not appear to be meeting children's mental health needs and may, in fact, serve to disempower individuals, families, and systems. Instead, we need to adopt an interdisciplinary, collaborative approach that results in a network of family-centered services that adequately support all students and improve long-term social–emotional and educational outcomes.

Three

Building Capacity Through Collaboration and Coalition Building

T hinking about how to create systemic change can be overwhelming at first. It seems like there are so many different aspects to consider, connections to make, and things to do. If it feels like it is too much for one person, that is simply because it is. As school psychologists, we have generally been trained in solitary forms of practice. We are the therapist, the examiner, the group facilitator, and the consultant. Moving toward a public health model requires us to move toward a new way of envisioning our role as a team member. As noted by Doll and Lyon (1998), it is "essential for schools and communities to align themselves in partnerships to foster resilience and capacity-building among high-risk students. Neither system has the resources to single-handedly interrupt recurrent cycles of risk" (p. 360).

Creating sustainable, systemic change is not an easy task and requires a great deal of time and effort. There are differing levels at which individuals and agencies can work together, ranging from simply communicating about one's efforts to developing a coalition. These different levels of working together are described in this chapter. From a public health perspective, a coalition with others who share similar goals and a common vision is necessary to promote positive change. This chapter highlights strategies for developing and supporting the work of collaborative teams that can address this expanded vision of mental health service provision.

LEVELS OF COLLABORATION

Consistent with the NASP Practice Model (2010), school psychologists "function as change agents, using their skills in communication, collaboration, and consultation to promote necessary change at the individual, student, classroom, building, and district, state, and federal level" (p. 5). This practice statement helps us to think about what we should be doing, but not necessarily with whom or how we should go about engaging in these different actions.

One of the initial steps is to define the level of collaboration that is needed and the different benefits that each can provide. True collaboration does not happen quickly; it is considered to be both a process and an outcome. Lawson (2003) outlined a developmental progression for collaboration which provides an effective tool for determining where your collaborative efforts are currently and where you might like them to be. The five levels or phases of collaboration are the following:

1. Connecting and communicating
2. Cooperation
3. Coordination
4. Community building
5. Contracting

The process is not always linear, although each step describes an increasing level of commitment on the part of the stakeholders.

Connecting and Communicating

At the first level, *connecting and communicating*, as a school psychologist, your activities include various levels of interaction (e.g., interpersonal, interprofessional) that help to build linkages between different organizations. This phase provides the foundation for collaboration and begins the process of increasing awareness of the language and culture of other entities. For example, to better understand a new mental health referral agency in town, you might contact the director and arrange a brief phone or direct interview to find out more about the process, the available resources, and strategies for how you can support families in accessing this resource. If you have been at your position for a few years, you have undoubtedly developed a number of community connections.

Cooperation

At the second level, *cooperation*, two or more organizations engage in a voluntary activity that builds the connection between the groups. With the combined efforts, trust develops and communication improves (Lawson, 2003). For example, you, as a school psychologist, might work with a therapist at a local mental health agency who is forming a parent support group. You might distribute flyers to potential family members and have the flyers available in the parent work room at school. This level of interaction is also common between school psychologists and individuals from local community agencies.

Coordination

At the third level, *coordination*, cooperation is enhanced because efforts are made by both entities to align their efforts. Using the same example of the parent support group, in addition to disseminating information about the group, the mental health agency representative and you might work together to identify goals for the group, strategies for reinforcing parent behaviors through school-based incentives, and special presentations by the school psychologist to help families support their children in school. This example describes two individuals coordinating their efforts; coordination refers also to the broader agencies working together. One of the benefits of coordination is that both partners begin to recognize and develop shared goals (Lawson, 2003).

Community Building

The fourth level of collaboration reflects a significant leap beyond coordination. This level is called *community building* and involves more formalized processes such as consensus building, greater awareness of mutual goals, and greater capacity for community action (Lawson, 2003). Community building is sometimes referred to as coalition building. Berkowitz and Wolff (2000) define a coalition as a "group involving multiple sectors of the community, coming together to address community needs and solve community problems" (p. 2). Community coalitions can help reduce fragmentation and duplication, provide better coordination, and monitor the quality of various programs. Beyond these immediate goals, coalitions can also foster trust, create a common forum to discuss issues, provide opportunities for community involvement, and, ultimately, raise community competence (Berkowitz & Wolff, 2000). Adelman and Taylor (2010) view coalitions as a type of collaboration involving different organizations that form "an *alliance* for sharing information and jointly pursuing cohesive policy advocacy for action in overlapping areas of concern" (p. 219).

Contracting

The final phase of collaboration reflects the most formalized agreement, *contracting*. At this level, one or more agencies engage in legal agreements, such as an interagency agreement or a university–school partnership, that outline the roles and responsibilities of each organization (Lawson, 2003). Although not part of the contract, Lawson (2003) noted that social agreements emerge from contracting and relate to the unwritten norms that develop between the different organizations that help to create and maintain trust.

It is important to recognize that contracting can occur without real partnership. For example, some schools have adopted a clinic within the school model where they contract with a local mental health agency for therapists to provide mental health services in the school setting. Too often, staff from these agencies are simply "co-located" rather than integrated into the school. As a result, there is little connection or coordination with school staff and only a small number of youth are able to access this resource (McMahon, Ward, Pruett, Davidson, & Griffith, 2000).

COLLABORATIVES AND COALITIONS

Collaboration involves many of the aforementioned activities, but it is also something more. Adelman and Taylor (2010) define comprehensive collaboration as a "way to weave together a critical mass of resources for moving forward" (p. 216). Collaboration is sustained, involves a shared vision, and members of the collaborative establish working relationships. The outcomes are broad and systemic and provide for better outcomes for children, families, schools, and communities. When a collaborative is formed, different agencies develop an infrastructure for working together to accomplish shared goals (Adelman & Taylor, 2010). We use the terms *collaboratives, coalitions*, and *community building* to refer to the act of bringing multiple agencies and community members together in a working relationship to address overlapping areas of concern. We recognize that practitioners are at various levels when it comes to building community partnerships and believe that movement toward any of these models is positive. Many of the key terms and actions discussed in the rest of this chapter are relevant to each of these models.

School psychologists are likely familiar with and have initiated some of the levels of collaboration mentioned earlier. It is also possible that your school or district has negotiated a contract with another agency (e.g., therapists-in-schools program, university–school partnership, interagency agreement) that you may participate in at some level. However, many have not taken these steps toward coalition building. As you think about your current or future efforts toward building a collaborative partnership, the form in the accompanying CD (3.1) can be used to guide your efforts. Additionally, it is important to consider some of the concepts associated with building community partnerships.

KEY COMPONENTS OF COLLABORATIVE PARTNERSHIPS

Building collaborative partnerships among school and community agencies is much more complicated than it might seem. There are differences in language, culture, priorities, legal and funding requirements, and general philosophies that can sometimes create fundamental gaps that are difficult to bridge. Too often, collaborative efforts fade away or are ineffective because there was not enough attention given to developing an infrastructure. There are many factors to consider when developing these collaborative relationships and we introduce the concepts of membership, building capacity, empowerment, process, and leadership to help define some of these issues. In Chapter 7, we will revisit these ideas to describe the types of activities that are important for coalitions, as well as ways of coordinating your efforts with local agencies.

Membership

Whether you looking at expanding your coordination with outside agencies or building a coalition, a key component is to identify major stakeholders and develop collaborative relationships with each group (Cowen et al., 1996). Before you begin to invite a group of potential stakeholders to join your interest group, it is important to speak with your building level administrator to ensure that you have support for your efforts. This conversation can also help clarify leadership issues, available resources, and any concerns that might interfere with your efforts further down the road. Once you have established that you have administrative support, your next step is to decide who to involve and how many members to invite.

If we were to ask you to name three key people you could talk to about a broad issue of concern (e.g., school dropout or some other key issue pertinent to your current academic setting), you could probably list more than a few school-based individuals as well as a community member or two who have taken a lead or voiced a strong opinion about this issue. That is a starting point to building a coalition: initiate a meeting with a few other individuals who share a common interest. Additionally, you can ask each of those individuals to invite one or two others who also share an interest. As your preliminary working group begins to identify additional potential members, you will need to keep a few key ideas in mind.

Generally, the more members you have, the more visible your efforts are, the more work you can accomplish, and the more you are able to empower members of the community. Within the schools, these stakeholder groups might include school administrators, general and special education teachers, related service personnel, family members, and students (Power, DuPaul, Shapiro, & Kazak, 2003). Outside of the school, community mental health providers, primary care physicians, after school programs, social services, and faith-based organizations might be important stakeholders to engage. The issue of concern may help pinpoint the voices that need to be at the table. For example, if your concern is increased gang activity, having a member from law enforcement or a gang unit makes sense. If the issue is related to the high number of young children who are expelled from preschool settings, you would want to invite operators of preschools, interagency council members, mental health team members who specialize in early childhood services, and parent advocates. As you are thinking about building this team, be sure to think outside of the school walls.

There can also be drawbacks to a large membership, such as greater difficulty in establishing trust between members, scheduling meetings, and ensuring clear and consistent communication across all members. When recruiting new members, personal contacts are usually the best method. To maintain your group membership, it is also important to help members see the benefits of becoming and remaining a member of your coalition. That is, people like to see progress, change, and hopefully, positive outcomes. If the group becomes bogged down in dissent and inaction, it is likely that many members will cease to remain involved. The goal of your coalition is to begin to work to build capacity.

Building Capacity

Building capacity refers to efforts that are "designed to enhance and coordinate human, technical, financial, and other organizational resources directed toward quality implementation of evidence-based, competence-building interventions through public education delivery systems" (Spoth, Greenberg, Bierman, & Redmond, 2004, p. 32). School psychologists possess many of the necessary skills for building capacity among a diverse group of stakeholders. For example, school psychologists have effective communication skills that allow them to work with individuals from a variety of backgrounds. Consultation and counseling skills can be put to good use when facilitating working groups in which individuals with differing perspectives must come together to develop a plan.

By implementing the steps of a problem-solving process, school psychologists can provide a framework to identify the needs, help establish goals, and decide on a potential plan to meet these goals. The basic elements of capacity building include public education, coordination of services, empowerment, and professional development for all of the stakeholders, including school administration, educational staff, mental health service providers, families, and community members. School psychologists are in a prime position to foster these efforts and help maintain programming (Nastasi, 2004). We provide detailed coverage of public education and professional development components in Chapter 7, as these will be outcomes of your work with your community partnership (as part of the Ecological Plan Implementation step). To build the capacity of all members of this partnership, empowerment practices must be present from the beginning.

Empowerment Practices

To be equal partners in any change effort, stakeholders need to be empowered. There are many different meanings for the word *empowerment* and these are generally based on a particular empowerment movement. Despite some differences, there are many points of agreement. Empowerment is active, participatory, and multi-level. Empowerment is a process that enables individuals to experience greater levels of control over their own lives (Rappaport, 1987; Segal, Silverman, & Temkin, 1995; Thompson et al., 1997). It is also important to consider some things that empowerment is not. It is not a top-down initiative, nor is it the simple distribution of knowledge. Finally, it is not empowerment to invite voices to the table and then not let them speak. Stakeholders must be able to act as partners in decision-making (Simon, 1994). As you are building your coalition and deciding on your processes (e.g., decision-making), consider the structure your group will use to make sure that everyone's voice will be heard and that all will be able to participate in making important decisions.

Empowerment requires a restructuring of the traditional relationships between students, parents, and professionals (Banyard & Goodman, 2009; Wolfendale, 1992). Part of this strategy includes sharing information between and among stakeholders, but it must also go beyond that. One of the most important goals of empowerment, as aligned with a public health model, is to enable others to achieve their goals—that is, to improve the self-efficacy of others. One example of this approach that is often seen within school settings is providing opportunities for parents to assist their own children as well as other parents in similar circumstances (Dunst, Trivette, & Johanson, 1994). Empowerment helps families to feel more connected to systems and more in control of what happens in their lives.

Levels of empowerment. Effective social movements and interventions require empowerment-related processes and outcomes across multiple levels of analysis (Zimmerman, 1995). Empowerment strategies can occur across three different domains. At the *psychological level*, empowerment is facilitated through choice, shared leadership, provision of opportunities for multiple and meaningful roles, and peer-based support systems. For example, the use of Professional Learning Communities (Darling-Hammond & Richardson, 2009) within schools is an important strategy for helping teachers to advance their knowledge and skills within the classroom by learning with and from their peers.

Empowerment strategies can also be directed at the *organizational level* by building on the psychological empowerment of members and improving organizational effectiveness to attain goals. At this level of analysis, we evaluate the structures and processes in place that help build on the members' skills and provide the needed supports to effect community change (Zimmerman, 1995). Within an educational system, this concept is referred to as school capacity (Cosner, 2009) and is defined as the organizational resources that support educational reform, teacher change, and positive student outcomes. Cosner (2009) described trust as one of the key resources for building school capacity. Through his interviews with 11 high school principals who were nominated for their skill in trust-building, he found that these school leaders built trust through activities such as increasing interaction times, creating new forums for interaction, and increasing the likelihood that trust would occur through these interactions (e.g., helping staff use interpersonal problem-solving effectively, introducing tasks that require interdependent problem-solving, using leadership and facilitation skills in interdependent groups).

At the broadest level, *community empowerment* involves individuals working together in an organized manner to deter community threats, improve quality of life, and generally facilitate citizen participation. Dowrick et al. (2001) described a comprehensive university–community partnership to implement interventions focused on literacy and aggressive interactions within elementary schools in an urban community. Neighborhood participants were able to move into roles of recruiting new members for the project, participating in data collection, monitoring and coaching one another, and participating in decision-making.

Evaluating empowerment practices. Use of an ecological model can provide a framework for evaluating the levels of empowerment that have been built into your coalition. For example, are you facilitating trust within your organizational system? Are all of your efforts designed to empower parents at the psychological level with no opportunities to enhance community empowerment? From a social justice perspective, empowerment strategies should be aimed at both the individual and community level: "Psychological empowerment cannot truly be achieved without actual access to resources and control—that is, political or social empowerment" (Banyard & Goodman, 2009, p. 273).

Some of the strategies that facilitate empowerment include collaborative planning, collaborative identification and recruitment of support systems in the environment (e.g., friends, community support services), education regarding legal issues and policy, and empowerment mentoring (Thompson et al., 1997). If parent empowerment is a learned behavior (as put forth by Thompson et al., 1997), then preparing parents in empowerment and providing a mentor to help them use their newly acquired skills may be an effective strategy for enhancing intervention outcomes and helping to sustain positive change.

We have long known that there is a strong relationship between family empowerment and treatment outcomes for youth in mental health care settings. Those caregivers who viewed themselves as more competent and knowledgeable had children who functioned better than those parents who felt less empowered (Resendez, Quist, & Matshazi, 2000). A recent study by Graves and Shelton (2007) indicated that as ratings of family empowerment increased (as measured by the Family Empowerment Scale), children's total problem behaviors decreased beyond the effect of the treatment program alone. These findings suggest that family empowerment may be an important mechanism of change in children's mental health programming.

Too often, we overlook student voice and empowerment in our efforts. Fullan and Stiegelbauer (1991) noted that adults "think of [students] as the potential beneficiaries of change [but they] rarely think of [them] as participants in a process of change and organizational life" (p. 170). Thus, empowerment efforts should also include students. McQuillan (2005) advocated for student empowerment as a means to help students remain engaged in their education, to assist in developing a complete picture of the effectiveness of reform efforts, and to help prepare youth for future responsibilities. As you move forward with your planning, consider how youth will be involved in planning, decision-making, and program implementation.

Process Components

As your coalition becomes more formalized and you determine a regular membership, you will need to work with the group to develop some kind of a structure and a process. When will you meet, how often, who will facilitate the meetings, who will set the agenda? These are all basic questions on which your group will need to make decisions. This leads to the next questions. What are the rules for decision-making? Does your group need to come to consensus, or is it enough to have a majority vote? Is a simple majority sufficient or should there be a "super" majority (e.g., 70%)? What are your basic operating procedures? Finally, how are you going to divide or delegate responsibilities to different members? It is ideal if all members participate in establishing the structure of your coalition.

In many ways, as a school psychologist, you deal with group process all of the time in your day-to-day work. For example, facilitating an individualized education program (IEP) meeting entails many of the same skills (e.g., acknowledging the input of others, reaching consensus, conflict resolution) that you would put to use in a larger group format. One of the key differences is that in any one school, there is an established culture or "way" of doing things. Part of the challenge for you will be to think about new ways of conceptualizing issues and approaching problems.

In their work related to the development of integrated health care, Short and Talley (1999) described a shift in traditional thinking about who we serve, how we serve them, and what the boundaries of our responsibilities are. For example, they propose that as school psychologists, we will need to change our perspective to seeing our students as intact units. In building a collaborative effort, it makes little sense to divide up individuals within a population and declare that the school will only deal with mental health issues that take place within the school, the family will deal with those that occur at home, and the community agency will provide services specific to the broader setting. Instead, it is much more effective to view students as having a set of needs and, although certain aspects of programming might be divided, the recipients are always viewed from a holistic perspective.

Furthermore, if we are going to provide comprehensive services, we will need to think more flexibly about when and where these services are provided (Short & Talley, 1999). That is, some "school-related" services may be provided in the community, and agency-based services might be more appropriately provided in the school setting. If the goal is to facilitate enhanced accessibility for all, then rigid definitions about where services are provided must be relaxed. The same is true of training and professional development. Rather than assuming that all services and training will take place onsite at the school, it is likely that other settings will also be the focus for some of your group's activities.

As you work with a relatively small group of individuals over a period of time, your process tends to fall into place fairly easily as everyone is following these unwritten guidelines or rules for interacting in group settings. When you bring together a larger group with members of different organizations, each with its own unique culture, misunderstandings and conflicts may arise. Further, as you involve parents who may not be familiar with school-based formal and informal patterns of group process, you are introducing yet another dynamic. There is no set of rules that will work for every situation, so it is best to set aside time during your first few meetings to ask the group about the process they would like to use. In general, you'll want to establish guidelines for inclusion of all voices, interaction processes (e.g., formal as in Robert's Rules of Order, or informal as in taking turns and raising one's hand), decision-making (e.g., open voting or secret, consensus or majority), and how to deal with conflict when it arises. It is important not to get bogged down in this process but also to be sure that you spend some time creating a general framework for the structure of your coalition.

The work of Nastasi, Moore, and Varjas (2004) details the Participatory Culture-Specific Intervention Model (PCSIM) that was developed specifically to build partnerships that will facilitate the design, implementation, and evaluation of mental health programs delivered in school settings. Nastasi et al. (2004) provide many helpful insights into developing these collaborative processes when working with diverse groups. Power, Dowrick, Ginsburg-Block, and Manz (2004) used a Participatory Intervention Model (an earlier form of PCSIM) to guide their work with community partners to teach literacy to young children in under-resourced, urban settings. Their case studies demonstrate the effectiveness of this type of model in engaging community partners and producing positive outcomes for students.

Leadership

The preceding conversation highlights the important issue of leadership. Who is going to facilitate this process? Who is going to call the meetings? Facilitate the meetings? Set the agendas? Attend to the communication and tasks between the meetings? Your coalition needs a leader or co-leaders. In the beginning, that person is likely to be you as the school psychologist, but you may share leadership with another individual in order to create a more inclusive process or simply to lighten the work load. As your coalition becomes more established, you may find that leadership rotates to other individuals within the group. One of the key aspects of your role is to work with your coalition to ensure that the group members share a common purpose or vision and that your leadership represents the whole coalition. Other aspects of this role include continued clarification of expectations and demonstrated follow-through.

To date, there has not been any research to demonstrate a direct link between collective forms of participation and student performance. However, in their review of several long-term projects focused on school reform, Datnow and Stringfield (2000) concluded that those schools that were most likely to institutionalize reform were those where educators at various levels worked together and shared goals. Similarly, researchers have suggested that collaboration is equally important for implementation and sustainability of innovative programming in community settings (McKay, Jensen, and CHAMPS Collaborative Board, 2010). Through their work, McKay et al. have identified five foundational elements of collaborative efforts: (1) shared goals, (2) distributed power, (3) recognition of skills and competencies in others, (4) communication, and (5) trust. Each of these components exists on a continuum and can be used by collaborative teams to monitor and evaluate their own efforts. An evaluation tool is provided on the accompanying CD (3.2) that can be used for this purpose.

CONCLUSION

Coalitions come together for a variety of reasons, including a mandate from an external source, new money (e.g., grant funded project), community crisis, or simply people of similar interests coming together to solve a problem. Collaboration at this level occurs when it becomes apparent, because of the complexity and interdependence of an issue, that no one entity can effectively address the issue on its own (Lawson, 2003). Creating sustainable, systemic change is not an easy task and requires a great deal of time and effort. One of your first steps in preparing to work from a public health model is to develop collaborative networks with others who share similar goals.

Contrary to previous clinical frameworks, school psychologists must work with stakeholders who share a common vision. School-based prevention programs that are directly linked to the central mission of the school and are aligned with goals to which school personnel are accountable are more likely to be successful (Greenberg et al., 2003). Using our skills as school psychologists, we can build coalitions that allow us to impact broader problems of practice. There is much that you can do in your school setting, working together with community supports, to help ameliorate both the occurrence and the negative effects of risk factors.

II

PUBLIC HEALTH PROBLEM-SOLVING MODEL

Never doubt that a small group of thoughtful, committed citizens can change the world. Indeed, it's the only thing that ever has.

—Margaret Mead

Now that you have a better understanding of a public health approach and the types of programming that could be delivered across the entire continuum, the chapters in this section will lead you through the steps of a Public Health Problem-Solving Model. Specifically, we detail strategies for determining which problems to address in your school, district, or community, deciding which intervention will best address sources of risk and supports, and evaluating your efforts.

At the individual student level, some form of a problem-solving model has become a prominent feature in the delivery of psychological services and the training of school psychologists (Reschly & Ysseldyke, 2002). This approach was derived from Bergan's (1977) behavioral consultation model, which included four sequenced phases similar to the following: (1) problem identification, (2) problem analysis, (3) plan implementation, and (4) evaluation of the implementation. With a public health model (Short & Strein 2007; Simeonsson, 1994), the appropriate units of analysis are population indicators, rather than individual student data. Accordingly, the problem identification, problem analysis, implementation, and evaluation phases of the problem-solving model are best addressed using techniques from epidemiology. We present the Public Health Problem-Solving Model, based on the work of Short and Strein (2007), as a basic tool for conceptualizing mental

Table II.1 Comparison of the Stages of the Problem-Solving
Process, Primary Prevention Implementation, and the Public Health
Problem-Solving Model

Public Health Problem-Solving Model	Problem-Solving Process	Primary Prevention Implementation
1. Problem Identification Through Applied Epidemiology (see Ch. 4)	Problem Identification	Operationalize target conditions and risk and protective factors.
2. Problem Analysis of Risk Factors and Protective Factors (see Ch. 5)	Problem Analysis	Generate risk models.
3. Defining Risk Factors and Protective Factors in Child–Environment Interactions (see Ch. 6)		Define risk in terms of child–environment transactions.
4. Ecological Plan Implementation (see Ch. 7)	Plan Implementation	Differentiate the characteristics of universal, selected, and indicated prevention.
		Propose temporal frames.
		Specify and prioritize primary prevention efforts.
5. Monitoring and Evaluating Outcomes (see Ch. 8)	Plan Evaluation	Monitor and evaluate prevention outcomes.

health services in schools and communities. This model provides an integration of primary prevention levels to yield comprehensive programs that are sensitive to the needs of multiple
classes and levels of clients. In our model, we blend the four
stages of problem solving: problem identification, problem
analysis, plan implementation, and plan evaluation with
Simeonsson's (1994) model for implementing primary prevention. Table II.1 provides a comparison of the stages, and a
checklist is provided on the CD (4.1).

With this model, you will be able to identify the greatest
needs in your specific setting, identify the variables that are
both contributing to and acting as buffers for your student
population, and design strategies for developing, implementing, and evaluating program outcomes. This section will outline the model in detail.

Four

Problem Identification Through Applied Epidemiology

The first stage of the Public Health Problem-Solving Model is called Problem Identification. To maintain a valence-free conceptualization of intervention target, we define a problem as "a question raised for inquiry, consideration, or solution" (*Merriam-Webster Dictionary*, 2008), rather than as a negative, pathological, or deficit state. This broader definition allows interventionists to address targets that are positive and need strengthening (e.g., academic achievement) as well as those that are negative and require remediation (e.g., substance abuse).

In the Problem Identification Stage, we look at the various factors that increase children's likelihood of developing a particular condition or problem (risk factors) or decrease that possibility (protective factors). This is much more complex than it seems. Children and their families develop and live in systems. They are influenced by these systems, and in turn they influence them. As described by Bronfenbrenner (1979), systems can be understood as existing in a somewhat hierarchical order based on the level of interaction and degree of impact on the individual. Common sources of risk and protective factors range from those that are found within the individual and expand out to peers, families, schools, and communities. Interventions to improve educational, health, and mental health outcomes can occur at any one or several of these levels. A comprehensive understanding of the interactions between systems and outcomes requires a careful consideration of each level, the relationships among factors and levels, and the overall relationships among predictive factors and outcomes. We must also consider that all of these interrelated elements

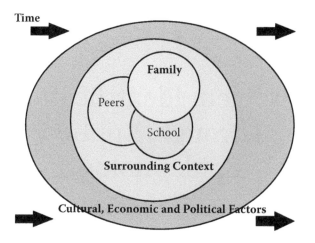

Figure 4.1 Individual in context.

develop over time, not least of which is the development of the individual(s) of interest. Figure 4.1 provides a graphic representation of this interactive relationship.

APPLIED EPIDEMIOLOGY

As stated in the introduction to Section II, our Public Health Problem-Solving Model utilizes an epidemiological approach to study risk and protective factors for populations. An epidemiological approach to problem identification focuses on population-wide indicators (e.g., curriculum based measurement [CBM] for an entire class, grade, or school) to identify *who* within the population (i.e., which subpopulations) has a problem, *when* such problems exist (time of year), *where* they exist (which grades, which teachers), and *why* they exist (identification of causes; Webb, Bain, & Pirozzo, 2005). Epidemiology has evolved and expanded from disease-specific outcomes to health, social, and behavioral dimensions of functioning. *Epidemiology* is defined by Last (1988) as "the study of the distribution and determinants of health-related states in specified populations, and the application of this study to control health problems" (p. 16). Epidemiology was originally defined as the study of disease, literally the study of epidemics; more modern versions encompass "health" broadly defined.

Applied epidemiology is the study of the distribution of health-related (or education- or mental-health-related) behaviors in a population in order to identify population-wide problems and develop effective population-wide interventions. This approach is differentiated from the original 19th-century model by "its insistence on explicitly investigating social determinants of population distributions of health, disease, and wellbeing, rather than treating such determinants as mere background to biomedical phenomena" (Krieger, 2001, p. 693). In school practice, applied epidemiology de-emphasizes learning disabilities, conduct disorders, or similar clinical diagnoses with etiologies within the person, and increases focus on sociocultural, familial, and environmental determinants of these problems. Further, this approach in school practice would examine disorders in the population with the intent of preventing them or lowering their incidence and prevalence, rather than addressing them in individual children. Table 4.1 shows a comparison of the Problem Identification Stage from a traditional versus applied epidemiological perspective.

The tools of epidemiology fall into two broad categories, both of which are covered in most psychological statistics courses: (1) data collection and summarization, and (2) inferential statistics. Data collection and summarization typically are used to provide information within the framework of *descriptive* epidemiology, whereas inferential statistics are the major implements of *analytic* epidemiology.

DESCRIPTIVE EPIDEMIOLOGY

As suggested by its label, the purpose of descriptive epidemiology is to provide objective information about a condition.

Table 4.1   Traditional Versus Applied Epidemiology Problem Identification

Traditional	Applied Epidemiology
• Collect data on individual students through standardized and nonstandardized psycho-educational assessment.	• Collect data on populations through surveillance systems or descriptive studies.
• Use data to inform special education placements or plan educational interventions.	• Use data to generate hypotheses about relationships among risk factors, protective factors, and outcomes.
• Devise interventions that focus on individual students.	• Devise community interventions to influence outcome for the entire population; interventions may be tailored to level of need, but all members of the population are considered.

School mental health professionals are familiar with practices that describe conditions as reliably and validly as possible. Indeed, much school-based practice involves just this type of activity, albeit at the level of the individual student instead of the population. In the same vein, descriptive epidemiology endeavors to define clearly the condition (*what*), the time frame for its occurrence (*when*), the setting or location of the condition (*where*), and the characteristics of individuals experiencing the condition (*who*). Whereas these dimensions historically have been applied to public health problems (e.g., AIDS, rubella, obesity), they apply just as readily to educational and mental health conditions (e.g., school completion, violence, learning disabilities).

For example, descriptive epidemiology applied to on-time school completion might define and count the number of students (*what*) in a school or community who finish high school within 4 years. These data might be gathered and reported over a several-year period (*when*) to provide information about trends in graduation. Particularly in large communities with multiple high schools, graduation rates may differ significantly depending on the high school. Accordingly, differential data can be gathered by high school (*where*) to provide information concerning where strengths and weaknesses exist in the system. Finally, even more specificity can be achieved by examining characteristics of students who complete or fail to complete school (*who*), including gender, socioeconomic status (SES), race and ethnicity, involvement in sports, and other characteristics. Taken together, these descriptive data provide a picture of the system regarding the issue of concern for the population of interest. (See CD 4.2 for an elementary school example.)

Typically, many of the measures in descriptive epidemiology are frequencies and describe two alternatives: alive or dead, case or control, exposed or unexposed, and so on. Applying this frame to education and psychology, an epidemiologist might count completers versus non-completers, students with learning disabilities versus those without, and so forth. Using frequency measures allows the calculation of several important statistics for epidemiological use, including ratios, proportions, and rates.

Ratios. Ratios refer to the relationship between two quantities, where the quantities are independent of each other and are expressed as a fraction or a decimal. For example, a pool with 360 females and 120 males yields a 360/120, or a 3:1, female-to-male ratio.

Proportions. Proportions are ratios in which the numerator is included in the denominator. Using the preceding example, 360 females in a total pool of 480 individuals (360 females + 120 males) yields a proportion of 360/480, or three quarters of the pool being female. Ratios and proportions are used in several ways in epidemiology, including calculation of risk ratios, odds ratios, proportionate mortality, and point prevalence.

Rates. Rates are special instances of proportions. Rates deal with the occurrence of an event in a population over time. They represent the number of cases or events in a given time period divided by the population at risk during that time period. Using the school completion example, if 1,917 of 2,500 students completed high school on time within the 4-year time frame, then the completion rate is 1917/2500, or .7668—typically multiplied by 100 to yield an on-time completion rate of 77%.

Morbidity Rates: Incidence and Prevalence

Although several types of rates are calculated in descriptive epidemiology, perhaps the most important rate for applying the public health model to school mental health is morbidity. Morbidity is a frequency measure that describes the presence of a characteristic (typically, a disease in the health domain), or the probability of its occurrence. In addition to overall measures of morbidity, specific measures of the characteristic can be calculated by race, gender, SES, or other important dimensions. In this way, differential risk rates can be determined for significant subgroups of the population. Morbidity rates can be calculated to yield two common statistics in epidemiology: incidence and prevalence.

Incidence rate. Incidence rate is a measure of risk and is the most commonly used measure for determining and comparing population characteristics. Incidence rate is defined as the probability of the onset or occurrence of any characteristic in a population in a given period of time. By using frequency rates rather than raw numbers of cases, assessors can control for differences in group size across populations and allow for cross-population comparisons. When one group exhibits a higher incidence rate than another group, that group is at higher risk of developing the characteristic than is the second group. Using a formula, incidence rate is

$$\text{Incidence rate} = \frac{\text{New cases in a time period}}{\text{Population in the same time period}} \times 10^n$$

Incidence rates only include new cases that appear during the time period relative to all persons susceptible to the condition. Generally, this number can represent the average population during the time period. Also, the time period must be specified to allow for comparison of incidence rates across populations or periods. Finally, the power of 10 used in the formula can be varied to make incidence statistics more meaningful (e.g., 472 new cases per 100,000 [10^5] or 4.7 new cases per 1,000 [10^3]).

Prevalence rate. Prevalence rate is similar to incidence rate but deals with *all* cases, instead of only *new* cases evident in a population during a specified time interval. Accordingly, the numerator in the prevalence rate formula includes both new and existing cases of the condition, whereas the denominator remains the population within a designated time period.

$$\text{Prevalence rate} = \frac{\text{New and existing cases in a time period}}{\text{Population in the same time period}} \times 10^n$$

Whereas incidence provides information about a disease or attribute's rate of change in the population, prevalence provides an index of severity or extensiveness of the disease or attribution in the population. Both measures can provide information about who needs services, where they are, and the time frame within which the problem or attribute occurs. However, incidence and prevalence rates are less useful for identifying causal paths and potential intervention targets— the why and how of the condition. These important activities require an analytic epidemiology approach.

ANALYTIC EPIDEMIOLOGY

Analytic epidemiology builds on findings from descriptive epidemiology to investigate possible causes of, and influences on, the problem or condition in the population. Figure 4.2 provides a diagram of the Analytic Epidemiology model. Using the descriptive results, the analytic epidemiologist develops hypotheses to explain the condition and then tests these hypotheses to yield empirical support for surmised correlates and influences. Because the inferential statistics used to develop and test these hypotheses essentially are the same as those included in all school psychology programs and many programs training other school mental health professionals,

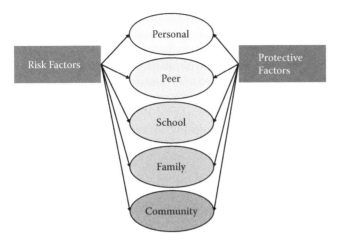

Figure 4.2   Building the model: Analytic epidemiology.

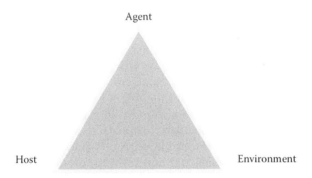

Figure 4.3   Epidemiological triad.

school practitioners should be familiar with much of the language and process of analytic epidemiology.

Three domains of investigation comprise the general framework for analytic epidemiology. These dimensions, called the Epidemiological Triad, are *Host*, *Agent*, and *Environment*, and are presented graphically in Figure 4.3. A basic assumption of analytic epidemiology is that disease can be explained by factors associated with one or more of these three dimensions. Analytic epidemiological studies often organize results along the lines of the triad.

Host. Host factors are intrinsic characteristics of individuals that cause them to be more susceptible, or resistant, to the condition. These factors can occur along social, physical, and psychological dimensions. For example, social characteristics of students, including SES and geographical location, may cause them to be more susceptible to obesity or depression. Physical attributes, including genetic makeup and anatomic structure also may contribute to vulnerability to obesity or depression. Psychological and behavioral factors, such as exercise and eating patterns, may explain even more of the variance associated with being overweight or depressed. All of these are characteristics of individual students. It is interesting to note that individual host characteristics traditionally have been the primary domain of psychological assessment; the epidemiological approach broadens assessment to acknowledge an ecological perspective.

Agent. Agent factors originally referred to infectious microorganisms, which had to be present for disease to occur. These agents included bacteria, viruses, and parasites and were seen as necessary but not sufficient causes of the disease. In the case of applied epidemiology, agent factors are less clear and often indistinguishable from environmental factors. Nonetheless, it is productive to examine causal factors as agents when clear and specific links can be demonstrated between such factors and the condition. For example, although not infectious and not actually a disease agent, maternal alcohol use is a causal agent for fetal alcohol syndrome. Agent factors can also be conceptualized in terms of likelihood that a problem or solution will be adopted. For instance, innovations that show relative advantage, that are compatible with other aspects of a social system, that are simple, that one can try before adopting, and that one can observe others using prior to adopting are more likely to be adopted (Rogers, 1995, 2002).

Environment. Environmental factors represent external determinants of a condition. Environmental factors are important in epidemiology in that they can affect the host, the agent, or the interaction between the host and the agent. Examples of environmental factors in public health epidemiology include crowding, sanitation, and other characteristics that serve to limit or spread disease. Environmental factors are similarly important in applied epidemiology, as they represent the primary targets of intervention to influence the incidence or prevalence of the condition in the population. For example, school failure may be partly explained by environmental factors such as school climate, teacher quality, parent behaviors, and availability of educational resources. In this example, understanding school failure in the population would require knowledge of the relative contributions of these and other environmental factors to the problem in order to plan interventions to influence its morbidity.

In behavioral and social epidemiology, environmental factors are often organized by their primary locus. Accordingly, school environmental factors might include classroom climate, instructional quality, or engaged time. Parent factors might include parenting style and parent education. Peer factors might deal with peer acceptance, number of peers, and peer behaviors. In this way, epidemiological researchers can develop understandable frameworks to guide monitoring, assessment, intervention, and evaluation. Short and his colleagues (Short & Brokaw, 1994; Short & Shapiro, 1993) developed a simple example of such a framework for conduct disorders, in which organization of dimensions of correlates of population problems and attributes can provide a useful heuristic for prevention practice and epidemiology. Additionally, such heuristics yields hypotheses concerning risk and protective factors associated with the problem or attribute that can guide intervention and evaluation.

DECIDING ON THE ISSUE OF CONCERN AND OPERATIONALIZING TARGET CONDITIONS

Although you could try to analyze incidence and prevalence rates for numerous problems, usually groups have decided that they wish to have certain issues addressed. These priorities are often established based on values, policy changes, or funding streams. As school-based practitioners, it is important that any target for change can show linkages to supporting students' K-12 academic achievement and readiness for post-secondary success. If there is more than one possible issue of concern, we would advocate that these be prioritized and addressed sequentially (or addressed by different groups) so as to promote chances of success and allow for more clear evaluation of impact. In discussing provision of individual services, Telzrow and Beebe (2002) argued the need to address "keystone behaviors," which they defined as pivotal behaviors that, if supported, would allow for students to flourish in multiple areas of development. This idea can be equally applied to a population-based public health problem-solving model. What specific issues need to be addressed to allow students to develop in multiple life areas? Discussions with multiple stakeholders will be important to make sure that your chosen interventions are aligned (and make explicit the linkages) to their priorities.

CONCLUSION

Practicing school mental health professionals can use descriptive epidemiology techniques combined with an analytic epidemiology approach to develop and evaluate empirically derived prevention programs. As a first step, incidence and prevalence of the population problem or attribute can be investigated by generating frequency rates of new cases and all cases within a time frame. Second, school practitioners can identify potential positive and negative correlates (risk and protective factors) from the literature and/or information at the site. Third, these relationships can be evaluated by gathering data on potential risk and protective factors and testing their association with incidence and prevalence of the problem or attribute in the population of interest. Fourth, interventions to influence significant risk and protective factors can be devised and implemented. Finally, changes in morbidity in relation to interventions can be evaluated. In this way, practitioners can make valuable, data-based contributions to remedying problems and promoting solutions to difficult issues in schools and communities.

Five

Problem Analysis of Risk Factors and Protective Factors

T he second stage in the problem-solving model is Problem Analysis. When applied to the Public Health Problem-Solving Model, this stage is expanded to identifying risk and protective factors. Ultimately, your knowledge of risk and protective factors in your school and community will be used to develop a prediction model, based on analytic epidemiology, that includes the target condition as well as risk and protective factors. In other words, we look at the various factors that increase students' likelihood of developing a particular condition or problem (risk) or decrease that possibility (protective).

The first step in this process is to develop a complex understanding of risk and protective factors; these concepts are much more complex than we might realize. Common sources of risk and protective factors range from those that are found within the individual and expand out to peers, families, schools, and communities. Interventions to improve educational, health, and mental health outcomes can occur at any one or several of these levels. A comprehensive understanding of the interactions between systems and outcomes requires a careful consideration of each level, the relationships among factors and levels, and the overall relationships among predictive factors and outcomes. Figure 5.1 shows the Problem Analysis Stage of the Public Health Problem-Solving Model.

IDENTIFYING AND UNDERSTANDING RISK FACTORS AND PROTECTIVE FACTORS

Understanding underlying factors and relationships among outcomes, individual characteristics, and environmental factors is a crucial step in developing policies and interventions to address them. The importance of these individual and

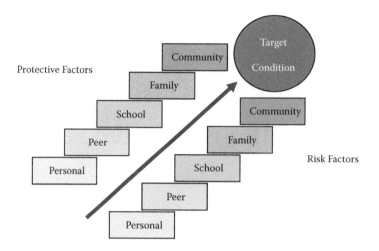

Figure 5.1   Problem analysis stage.

environmental characteristics, called risk and protective factors, lies in the extent to which they are related to outcomes
we want to influence and the extent to which we can alter
them to affect these outcomes.

Risk Factors

Risk factors have been defined as individual or environmental
hazards that increase vulnerability to negative developmental
behaviors, events, or outcomes (Masten, 2001; Werner & Smith,
1982). Because a risk factor indicates a higher probability that
a disorder will develop, it must predate the development of
the disorder. Risk factors can be fixed (e.g., sex, race, genetic
history) or they can be fluid (e.g., neighborhood, school, peer
group). One important concept to establish when considering
risk factors is the degree to which it is causal or associated.
For example, heavy drug use may cause increased expression
of schizophrenia in some vulnerable individuals (Semple,
McIntosh, & Lawrie, 2005). Conversely, an inability to visually
track moving objects with smooth eye movements is associated with the later development of schizophrenia but is not
thought to cause it (Ross, Radant, Heinlein, & Compagnon,
2003). Therefore, when developing an intervention plan to
reduce the likelihood that a group of vulnerable individuals
will develop schizophrenia, we would target a reduction in
heavy drug use rather than eye movement. However, as we
know that smooth eye movement difficulties increases the

probability of developing schizophrenia, increased screening for schizophrenia symptoms would be indicated for this group. In other words, we want to target the causal factors and monitor individuals with the associated ones.

One of our ultimate goals in identifying risk factors is to identify those that are both malleable and potentially causal to specific disorders. Unfortunately, this is a difficult task because the relationship between risk and positive and/or negative outcomes is incredibly complex and difficult to untangle. Mental health disorders can come about for many different reasons (e.g., risk factors) and via any number of routes (e.g., internal, familial, community). Furthermore, a particular vulnerability may not develop into a disorder when it occurs in the context of a protective factor. That is, the protective factor may mediate or act as a "buffer" between the individual and the risk. A related concept is that certain environmental factors are not always uniformly negative or positive in their effects. For example, we often think of harsh, authoritarian parenting practices as leading to negative outcomes for children. However, Deater-Deckard and Dodge (1997) have shown that although this type of parenting predicts antisocial behavior in White, middle-class children, it does not have the same child outcomes in African American families.

Equifinality and multifinality of outcomes. Two additional key concepts in the study of risk are equifinality and multifinality (Cicchetti & Rogosch, 1996). In *equifinality*, multiple pathways may lead to a common outcome. For example, aggressive behavior might result from physical abuse, injury to the frontal lobes, coercive parenting approaches, or an inherited tendency toward disinhibition (Raine, Brennan, & Mednick, 1997). Any one of these factors on its own, or two or more occurring together, could result in a higher risk of aggressive behavior. The second principle, *multifinality*, refers to the idea that a particular risk factor (e.g., maternal depression), might result in any number of adverse outcomes (Cicchetti & Rogosch, 1996; Durlak, 1997). Most importantly, we must keep in mind that presence of a risk factor does not mean that a negative outcome is inevitable. As strengths-based research has shown, individual competence is a multidimensional, dynamic, and ongoing process (Leadbeater, Schellenbach, Maton, & Dodgen, 2004).

Categorizing risk factors. There are several ways of organizing our thinking about risk factors. For example, some researchers have differentiated among risk factors depending on the malleability of those factors. This organization can be seen in the model proposed by Kraemer et al. (1997), where risk factors were organized in the following manner: (a) fixed factors that cannot be changed; (b) variable factors that can be changed but without apparent or immediate effect on outcomes; and (c) causal factors that can be changed and, when they are, improve outcomes. These categories are of special relevance for prevention practices, since large numbers of fixed risk factors have been identified, but relatively few of these inform efforts to create positive change. Risk factors can also be conceptualized from different levels or contexts, consistent with the ecological model presented in Chapter 2; these levels might include the individual, family, peers, school, and community.

Risk factors in context. Research on risk factors for mental disorders from the Institute of Medicine (IOM; 1994), the Report of the Surgeon General (U.S. Department of Health and Human Services, 1999), and the World Health Organization (WHO; 2005) has revealed sets of factors that are common to many disorders. As noted, they can be grouped by the contextual level of risk. At the individual level, a student might present with certain neurophysiological deficits, a difficult temperament, chronic illness or pain, below average intelligence, *in utero* exposure to substances, low birth weight, and/or sensory disabilities or organic handicaps (IOM, 1994; WHO, 2004). In and of themselves, these factors may present challenges for the individual, but more important is the interaction between the individual and the environment. A child that struggles to stay on task and follow classroom rules may struggle in an environment marked by an extremely rigid structure, low tolerance for off-task behavior, and a teaching style that relies heavily on lecture. Conversely, the same child might thrive in an environment that is structured but flexible, and where much of the learning occurs through project-based, hands-on learning activities.

Therefore, it is also important to consider the microsystemic variables of school and family and the risk factors present in those contexts. Using the same body of research mentioned previously, the risk factors associated with the microsystem level include academic failure, exposure to violence, child maltreatment and neglect, severe family discord or disorganization, low socioeconomic status, overcrowding or large family size, paternal criminality, and maternal mental illness. At a broader level, the exosystem is made up of those community variables that might play a role in the child's risk but may or may not directly impact the child on a regular basis. For example, residence in an area with social disorganization and poor schools is considered a risk factor for a number of negative outcomes, including antisocial behavior and school dropout.

Application of risk factors in epidemiology. When risk factors are identified through epidemiological research, preventive approaches can be developed to modify these factors. Rutter (1987) described five ways to reduce the stress of a risk factor: (1) Help individuals change the ways that they experience a risk factor (e.g., use coping strategies), (2) reduce or change individuals' exposure to the risk factor (e.g., increase parental monitoring around antisocial peers), (3) interfere with negative chain reactions (e.g., harsh parenting can lead to increasingly oppositional behavior which in turn leads to increased conflict), (4) strengthen protective factors, and (5) introduce turning points that change an individual's context and offer new opportunities (e.g., move to a new school or neighborhood).

Risk factors can also help us to identify populations that may benefit from interventions (e.g., children whose parents are divorcing; NRC & IOM, 2009). For example, based on extensive research, the IOM (1994) listed five risk factors for depression: (1) having a close biological relative with a mood disorder; (2) having a severe stressor such as divorce, job loss, traumatic experience, or learning disorder (in children); (3) having low self-esteem or low self-efficacy; (4) being female; and (5) living in poverty. Given this information, if we were deciding on a potential group of recipients for prevention programming related to depression, we could identify students who might benefit based on some of these risk factors. For example, children of parents with mood disorders are a good target for preventive programs because these children are likely to have genetic and psychosocial risk factors for depression.

In the best case scenario, we would know the exact risk as well as the pathway for a specific outcome so that our intervention could be targeted. However, that is not always possible. As we described earlier in the chapter, one risk factor might be associated with any number of different outcomes, or several different risk factors might be associated with the same outcome. Therefore, rather than attempting to track the potential outcome of each of these risk factors, we have identified some of the most common risk factors found in the literature as well as the context (see Table 5.1; for a more complete table organized by specific disorder, risk factors, and developmental stage, see http://www.nap.edu/openbook.php?record_id=12480&page=522).

Table 5.1 Social Ecology of Mental Health Risk Factors

Context	Risk Factors
Individual	Comorbid disorder (internalizing or externalizing)
	Genetic risk/vulnerability
	Illness
	Difficult temperament, poor self-regulation, impulsive sensation seeking, behavior problems
	Depressogenic cognitive style
	Behavioral inhibition and anxiety sensitivity
	Early puberty
Family	Stressful family environment (e.g., divorce, single parent)
	Use of corporal punishment, harsh parenting/lax rules
	Poverty
	Abuse (physical, sexual, emotional)
	Parental mental illness
	Parental substance abuse
	Maternal inattention
	Parental death
Peers	Delinquent peers
	Poor peer relations
	Victimization/bullying
School	Lack of bonding to school
	Poor academic achievement
Community	Neighborhood crime
	Residential instability
	Availability of illegal activities/substances
	Norms, values, and beliefs of residents (e.g., in relation to substance use, crime)

Source: Abramson et al., 2002; Biederman et al., 1993; Cohen, Brook, Cohen, Velez, & Garcia, 1990; Crews et al., 2007; Hawkins, Catalano, & Miller, 1992; Mayes & Suchman, 2006; McMahon, Grant, Compas, Thurm, & Ey, 2003; Melhem, Walker, Moritz, & Brent, 2008; Roosa, Sandler, Gehring, Beals, & Cappo, 1988; Sandler, Wolchik, Braber, & Fogas, 1986; Wyman, 2003.

Protective Factors

Because many risk factors cannot be changed, it is important to look at those variables that reduce risk or serve as protective factors against unchangeable risks. School-based prevention and youth development programs are most effective when they target students' personal and social assets, help connect them to others, and facilitate connections to the community (Eccles & Appleton, 2002; Greenberg et al., 2003). Protective factors are those variables in the individual, family, or community that are thought to reduce the likelihood of developing negative or problematic outcomes (NRC & IOM, 2009). Similar to risk factors, protective factors can be present in the individual, family, institutions, or communities.

Sometimes the term *protective factor* is mentioned in association with resilience. *Resilience* can be defined as better than expected outcomes, or competence, in the presence of risk factors (Luthar, Cicchetti, & Becker, 2000; Werner & Smith, 1982). Other definitions include an interactive component where protective factors reduce the negative impact of a specific risk factor (Luthar, 2006). Protective factors are thought to mediate or act as a buffer to environmental hazards. For example, living in a dangerous neighborhood may place a child at risk for any number of negative outcomes; however, having a close relationship with a caring adult may act as a protective factor and reduce the chances that the individual experiences any of the negative outcomes usually associated with that type of environment.

Protective factors and resiliency represent a relatively new contribution to preventive theories and have not been studied to the same extent as risk factors. However, several protective factors for mental health have been identified: positive temperament (e.g., adaptability, autonomy), above average intelligence, early cognitive stimulation, literacy, physical exercise, a feeling of mastery and control, social competence, positive attachment and early bonding, a close relationship with a supportive adult, social support of family and friends, and attending well-organized, achieving schools (IOM, 1994; WHO, 2005). Much like risk factors, protective factors can be more or less malleable. For example, in her comprehensive review of developmental resiliency research, Werner (2006) identified intelligence, temperament, and emotional reactivity as important attributes that help an individual to withstand adversity. Unfortunately, none of these characteristics is easily changed. Other factors, such as positive self-concept, achievement motivation, internal locus of control, impulse control, and planning and foresight, are more readily modified and may provide us with an avenue for developing effective interventions (Brehm & Doll, 2009). A list of common protective factors is provided in Table 5.2.

Table 5.2 Social Ecology of Mental Health Protective Factors

Context	Protective Factors
Individual	Intelligence
	Lower cortisol reactivity
	Able to accomplish age-appropriate tasks
	Self-reflection, self-understanding, higher internal control
	Problem-solving and coping abilities
Family	Positive family environment
	Effective parenting
	Adequate monitoring and supervision
	Positive relationship with an alternative caregiver
Peers	Engaged in relationships that are positive and reciprocal
	Social support
School	Supportive individual at school
	Academic achievement
Community	Stable neighborhood
	Community resources

Source: Beardslee & Podorefsky, 1988; Bolger & Patterson, 2003; Davies, Sturge-Apple, Cicchetti, & Cummings, 2007; Grant et al., 2006; Pina et al., 2008.

RISK FACTORS AND PROTECTIVE FACTORS SUMMARIZED

It is compelling to conceptualize risk and protective factors in a linear fashion. That is, if we identify a malleable risk factor, provide an intervention to change the individual's exposure or experience of that risk, we will then have averted some negative outcome. Of course it is not that simple. However, that is the general idea behind our efforts to identify risk and protective factors. At this point, we know more about risk factors than protective factors. In many instances, risk factors and protective factors represent the same variables; the degree of risk or protection is based on the direction in which it is scored (e.g., low academic achievement vs. adequate academic performance; Crews et al., 2007; Luthar, 2006). (See CD 5.1 for a sample form for analyzing risk and protective factors.) The following points summarize some of our current thinking on risk and protective factors (NRC & IOM, 2009).

- Risk and protective factors operate at multiple levels (e.g., individual, family, peers, school, and community).
- Both risk factors and protective factors are highly correlated and their effects are cumulative.

- Risk and protective factors can be general to many different types of outcomes or specific to certain disorders. Some risk factors are specific to gender and age.
- Risk and protective factors interact and influence one another across time. For example, early risk may be moderated by a protective factor leading to lower levels of risk as a child grows.

APPLYING OUR KNOWLEDGE OF RISK AND PROTECTIVE FACTORS: GENERATING RISK MODELS

Selecting Interventions

Although you likely won't be developing your own interventions, understanding the underlying theory for potential programs will assist your team in the decision-making process. Only your team can understand the unique circumstances of your setting. You may be at a suburban high school where middle-class to affluent students attend and the overall academic achievement is above the state average. If the students in your school are experiencing high levels of depression and suicidal ideation, programs that have been developed to address the risk factors of negative community influences and other factors potentially associated with lower socioeconomic situations may not be an appropriate fit for your potential participants. In this instance, you'd want to look for a program that was designed to address more intrapersonal and interpersonal risk and protective factors. An understanding of the risk and protective factors that are specific to your district or setting helps to guide you in selecting the most appropriate programming.

Selecting Recipients

Another key reason for identifying risk and protective factors is for the purpose of selecting potential recipients of your preventive interventions. Expanding on the previous example, having a parent who is depressed is a significant risk factor for children developing depression. Therefore, children of parents who are depressed or have mood disorders would be appropriate candidates for a selective intervention that targeted problem-solving and coping with difficult circumstances, and perhaps included a psychoeducational component that helped children better understand depression. In a school setting, it might be difficult to access parental depression data;

therefore, you might look to some of the other risk factors, for example, having experienced a severe stressor and having low self-esteem. The other two, being female and living in poverty, may not be helpful in narrowing down your potential participants as one would clearly represent half of your school population and, depending on the demographics of your setting, living in poverty may also include too many, or too few, potential participants. Once you've narrowed down the risk factors that you will focus on, the next step will be to survey your students. Guidelines for identifying levels of services for students with different needs are provided in CD 5.2. Strategies for conducting needs assessments are addressed in the next chapter.

Building Logic Models

A third reason for identifying risk and protective factors is for use in developing a logic model. The logic model will assist you in planning, designing, implementing and evaluating your program. A logic model is a tool that helps organize our thinking and provides a visual representation of our ideas. Logic models show how different elements of your project are related to one another and the types of outcomes that can expected as a result of your intervention or program (Knowlton & Phillips, 2009). Development of a logic model is described in the next chapter.

CONCLUSION

Identifying and targeting specific risk and protective factors associated with negative outcomes is a relatively new science and has a long way to go. Fortunately, because there is so much overlap in the various risk and protective factors, designing interventions that reduce specific risk factors or strengthen certain protective factors will likely be effective in addressing several conditions. For example, we know that child abuse is a risk factor for a variety of mental health disorders. If we implement solid programming that reduces the incidence of child abuse and enhances the resiliency of children in difficult home conditions, we are likely reducing the incidence of a number of negative outcomes. Using currently available information on risk and protective factors, we can design interventions to prevent mental problems and to identify those youth who will receive the greatest benefit from these supports.

Six

Defining Risk and Protective Factors in Child– Environment Interactions

One of the first steps in understanding a problem is to clearly define it as described in Chapter 4. Sometimes there is a tendency to plunge headlong into solving a problem without really understanding all of its complexities. In addition to researching your issue and knowing the facts, you want to gain as much expertise as possible (Berkowitz & Wolff, 2000). Melton (2005) cautions that you want to pay careful attention to the research and stay within the parameters of what is known.

A second caution is to ensure that the problem you have identified is amenable to change. For example, if you attempt to define a problem as "more than 60% of the children in this school come from single-parent households," you are likely to feel defeated before you even begin because this issue is not readily changed. In fact, Hoefer (2006) proposes defining a problem as a "situation that should be changed and can be changed" (p. 55). Therefore, you would want to dig deeper to identify what it is about that situation that creates a problem. The resulting problem definition can then be adapted to something that can be changed. For example, changing the problem statement to "we have a number of students who are not supervised for 2 to 3 hours each day after school because their parent is working" lends itself to potential solutions. (See CD 6.1.)

With a good understanding of risk factors and protective factors, you are ready to move to the next step in the process, which is applying that knowledge in a step-by-step process that will assist you in decision-making and program development. When applying your knowledge of risk factors and protective factors to an identified problem or concern, it is important to find the balance between overly simple explanations and spending too much time trying to find one specific causal factor. Instead, you'll rely on a combination of needs assessments, correlational findings from the literature, and the input of your stakeholders. Once you've decided on the issue you'd like to address (e.g., school bullying, high levels of teen pregnancy, as identified through an applied epidemiological approach), your next step is to use your understanding of the important risk and protective factors associated with that issue to begin your decision-making process. The previous chapter outlined many of the identified risk and protective factors established in the literature, but you'll also want to use data from your setting to establish factors that are unique to your setting.

IDENTIFYING AND MEASURING RISK FACTORS AND PROTECTIVE FACTORS

Descriptive epidemiology helps you clarify your identified problem, but analytic epidemiology allows you to make decisions about how you'll address the issue. What risk and protective factors are associated with this specific area of concern? Which of these are causal versus associative? Which ones can be modified? You will want to build a model that includes the target condition and the related risk and protective factors. Information to complete this task can be gleaned from surveying the research literature, using your own professional knowledge of the population, and listening to important participant informants. Issues such as bullying and victimization, academic underachievement and failure, poor peer relationships, violence, and substance use are all risk factors that are associated with neighborhoods and schools (NRC & IOM, 2009).

Fortunately, many organizations have already carried out the work of identifying risk and protective factors associated with some of the most common negative outcomes in youth (e.g., school dropout, teen pregnancy, violence). Information about these organizations and Web site links are provided on the CD (6.2). We have provided a brief description of some of these organizations and the types of resources that they provide. This list represents just a few of the resources that are free and readily available. We encourage you to look for additional resources that will facilitate screening and assessment at your own site.

The Substance Abuse and Mental Health Services Administration (SAMHSA) has developed a survey, a prevention manual, and a community leader's guide that can help communities identify a broad range of risk and protective factors in their youth and implement effective programs to address concerns. The Communities That Care Youth Survey can be administered in 50 minutes to 6th- through 12th-grade students and used to help identify youth who might benefit from more targeted interventions. Additionally, there is an accompanying prevention guidebook that provides information on more than 50 programs that have evidence to support their use with students from different developmental levels, to address specific risk and protective factors in different domains (e.g., individual, family, school, community) and at different levels (e.g., universal, selective, indicated). All resources associated with the Communities That Care program (e.g., survey, prevention guide, leader's manual) are available for free on their Web site.

The Centers for Disease Control and Prevention (CDC) has also developed a youth risk survey (Youth Risk Behavior Surveillance System [YRBSS]) that is used to monitor the degree to which youth are engaging in specific behaviors that are associated with health risks. Questions regarding seatbelt and helmet use; exercise; use of sun protection; tobacco, alcohol, and substance use; engaging in sex; and perceived safety and aggression (e.g., fighting, carrying a weapon) are all part of this survey. The information is used for a variety of purposes, but the current focus for the CDC is to monitor the degree to which the United States is meeting its goals for the Healthy People 2010 initiative. The two overarching goals for this initiative were to increase quality and years of healthy life and eliminate health disparities. On a positive note, the rate of health-risk behaviors among high school students has decreased. Unfortunately, a substantial percentage of youth continue to engage in behaviors that place them at risk for early mortality (e.g., carrying a weapon, riding in a car with someone who has been drinking) (Eaton et al. 2010). Individual states and counties have used the data for such purposes as developing a health curriculum and programming within educational settings or using the information to support community-based programs to increase physical activity (CDC, n.d.).

If your state or county uses these types of surveys, it may be relatively simple to access the data for your community in order to develop a better understanding of the kinds of risk and protective factors that are present. This information may also be helpful in targeting additional problem areas of which school personnel may not be aware. If this type of data is not collected, it may be helpful to approach your county health department to determine whether they might be interested in administering this type of survey. For example, many counties are now focusing on issues related to childhood obesity. The YRBSS may be useful as a monitoring device for obesity-tracking purposes, and other components (e.g., suicidal ideation and attempts, perceived threat at school) could be extremely helpful for your efforts.

An alternative, also offered through the CDC, is the School Health Index: A Self-Assessment and Planning Guide. This simple self-assessment tool consists of eight modules that cover topics such as nutrition, school safety, physical activity, health services, health promotion, counseling, psychological and social services, and family involvement. The self-assessment is completed by a group of school stakeholders such as the principal, nurse, school counselor and school psychologist, as well as parents and community representatives (e.g., health department, community mental health, American Cancer Society). After responding to the series of discussion questions for each module, the group completes an overall score card for the school, chooses their top five priorities for action, and then uses the free materials (e.g., training modules, meeting agendas, ideas for team members) provided on the Web site, or from other sources, to begin addressing their goal areas.

The Collaborative for Academic, Social, and Emotional Learning (CASEL) also lists a number of needs and outcome assessments that are available for free on their Web site. These instruments vary in the range of behaviors that they assess. Most are focused on a broad range of health behaviors (e.g., California Healthy Kids Survey, YRBSS). However, if your team were interested in measuring a very specific type of outcome, the Child Trends Youth Development Outcomes Web site is an excellent source for these focused measures. On this site, a list of possible outcomes that you might be interested in measuring (e.g., Parent–Child Relationship, Mental Health, School Engagement) is provided. Then, for each, a brief review of why it is important, a list of available measures including where they can be accessed, relevant citations in the literature, the advantages/disadvantages of the measure, and the cost are all listed in a concise manner. Other resources include the Center for the Study and Prevention of School Violence, Center for Mental Health in Schools, and Annie E. Casey Foundation.

By familiarizing yourself with these Web sites, you can quickly access existing assessments that can help you and your team gather important information about potential problem areas as well as the types of risk and protective factors that are unique to your setting and your student population. On the CD (6.3), we have provided a Risk Factors Estimation Form that can be used by stakeholders to provide their input on perceived risk factors and the percentage of the population impacted. These resources can save a substantial amount of time because you do not have to put your efforts toward test development and can instead focus on the problem-solving aspect of selecting and implementing the most appropriate and effective preventive interventions.

CREATING AND REFINING YOUR LOGIC MODEL

Too often, schools adopt fragmented programming that is not theoretically driven, is short term, and is not connected to the mission and culture of the school (Greenburg et al., 2003). By creating a logic model that explains the target condition in terms of risk factors and protective factors, you are better able to evaluate the specific areas where you would expect to see change.

Components of a logic model. A program logic model provides a detailed diagram that outlines all the various components of your program (Frechtling, 2007). The model begins with the *resources* or *inputs* that are necessary for the program to function. This component might include a mental health person to deliver the curriculum, curriculum materials, participants, a place to meet, incentives for attendees, and so forth. The second piece of the model includes the *activities*, or actions, that your team will take to carry out each strategy. If you were delivering a group to participants who were at risk for a particular problem, the activities would include the delivery of the group and other strategies you might use. For example, perhaps in addition to your group to help reduce aggressive behaviors, you're also helping teachers in your school to become more aware of low levels of aggression or cyber bullying and strategies for reducing this behavior among students.

The final pieces of a logic model include *outputs* and *outcomes*. *Outputs* are the products or direct *outcomes* of doing the specified activities. That is, these components might address the number or percentage of teachers who begin implementing a specific program after having been trained in its use. *Outcomes* refer to the hypothesized effects that the *outputs* will have on the systems and individuals targeted. Using the previous example, the *output* would be the number of teachers who began implementing a specific program in the classroom (e.g., Good Behavior Game), and the *outcome* would be students demonstrating decreased levels of aggressive behavior. It is important to separate these two components as the separation highlights the importance of ensuring that the recipients of the activities were able to access and use the information or training. The *outputs* must be in place in order to meet the expected *outcomes*.

Outcomes are often divided into short-term, medium-term, and long-term *outcomes*. As our work is school based and schools are in the business of educating students, we argue that short-term *outcomes* should include the effects on students and systems change for the school or district. The medium- and long-term *outcomes* should address academic success, as well as the intended mental health outcomes. To these standard elements of a logic model, we have added an encompassing box that represents the *Environmental Elements and Context*. It can be important to list the resources and constraints under which the intervention design and implementation will occur. Next, consider the risk and protective factors that appear to be present in the environment and that are related to the issue. Be sure to consider factors at various levels (e.g., individual, family, school, and community) to make your model as complete as possible. Figure 6.1 provides an overview of the components of a logic model (described in more detail in Chapter 8).

Continuing to develop and refine the logic model. At this point, you can develop a "pre" logic model to initiate discussions and to help you identify where you need to collect more information. After reviewing the data from your stakeholders and your needs assessment, do you need to modify your targeted issue, how it should be addressed, or what you expect to be the outcomes? If so, revise and clarify your logic model. As you

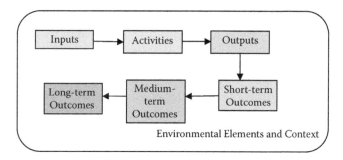

Figure 6.1 Logic model components.

continue into implementation of the *activities*, it is important to continue to return to your logic model and revise as needed.

Example: Initial development of a logic model. Once you have measured the risk factors and protective factors in your own site, determine the degree to which the hypothesized risk and protective factors are playing a role in the targeted condition. For example, there is increasing concern in your school and in the community that students are beginning to use substances at earlier ages, and their attitudes seem to reflect an acceptance of this use (and abuse). In fact, from your survey forms, you find that the students in your school are using at higher rates than the national average and that they are using at earlier ages than you were aware. It seems to have moved beyond the typical adolescent experimentation, and negative outcomes are being reported (e.g., higher rates of tardiness and increased truancy, students caught with alcohol on campus, increased rates of fighting at after school events). Therefore, your team decides that the targeted issue is to decrease substance use among students in your school district. Since attitudes toward substance use, and in some cases substance use itself, start in childhood, you want to coordinate your efforts across your feeder schools, not just at the high school level.

Based on the review of the literature, you know some of the individual risks for substance use are poor impulse control, sensation seeking, antisocial and problem behaviors, and early substance use. Family risk factors include permissive parenting, inadequate supervision, parent–child conflict, parents holding a favorable attitude toward substance use, and modeling from older siblings. School risk factors include school failure, low engagement with school, peer attitudes that support use, a deviant peer group, and alienation from peers. In the community, accessibility and availability, extreme poverty, and laws/norms that tolerate use are all risk factors. Some of the family-level protective factors for substance abuse include a warm, nonconflictual relationship with parents, adequate supervision, and parents who do not model drug use (NRC & IOM, 2009). At school, healthy peer groups and engagement with school are considered to be protective factors. Communities that enforce laws related to cigarette and alcohol sales and provide positive role models also have lower levels of substance use.

Clearly, there is no way to address all of these risk factors. Therefore, you use the data from your surveys to determine which factors are most relevant in your setting. Perhaps there are a few students who are at high risk because of their long history of behavioral problems and sensation seeking, but this does not seem to be the reason for the overall high rate of substance use. Instead, you decide to focus on other risk factors. Your school is located in a lower middle-class neighborhood where both parents in most families work and you know inadequate supervision is a problem; however, you decide that there is not a lot that can be done from the family's perspective. Instead, your group decides to provide more after school and community activities, where young people in the community will be more closely supervised. Your focus will be on building refusal skills in students (to resist peer influence). You want to build awareness of social influences on substance use and help change the "norm" around substance use; you want to generally build the social resistance skills among the students in your schools; and you want to work with community leaders to make sure that laws prohibiting sales to minors, minors in possession, and community curfew hours are upheld. Although it is not a central focus of your intervention, you plan to send home information and tips for parents on how to talk to their children about substance use, strategies for monitoring and supervising adolescents, and to help parents be aware of the efforts that the school is taking to reduce substance use among students.

With these clear ideas in mind, your next step is to select a program or programs that will support your efforts. Using some of the resources from the Web sites listed earlier, you know the LifeSkills Training program (Botvin, 2000; Botvin & Kantor, 2000) is a commonly used substance abuse prevention program that is considered a model program by the Blueprints for Violence Prevention and the Surgeon General's Youth Violence Report (NRC & IOM, 2009). The LifeSkills Training program focuses on resisting social influences and increasing social competence in middle and high school students. This curriculum is provided to entire classrooms and is initially delivered across 15 45-minute sessions. In the second year, students are provided with 10 class sessions, and in the third year, 5 classroom booster sessions. Your team decides that this universal approach is most appropriate because of the pervasiveness of the issue.

Your team also recognizes that it is important to integrate mental health promotion activities to help youth feel connected, to build stronger relationships with their family and community, and to increase the students' sense of self-efficacy and determination. Using information from Catalano et al. (2004), you decide to incorporate strategies that are consistent with positive youth development. Specifically, you want to provide students with opportunities for prosocial involvement, foster prosocial norms and behaviors, and recognize students' positive behaviors. A positive youth development program that has incorporated these components and has been shown to reduce substance abuse is Project Northland (Perry et al., 1993, 2000). In this program, students participated in classroom curriculum around substance abuse prevention, planned and participated in alcohol free events at their schools and family nights, and engaged in community activism. Your team decides to try some of these elements rather than adopting the entire program and works to involve as many students as possible in developing after school programs that focus on planning alcohol-free events, family nights, and service learning projects (e.g., raising funds for a local animal shelter, volunteering, refurbishing bicycles that can be donated to children). Your goal is to involve as many students as possible in these activities in order to establish norms around leisure activities without substances, giving to one's community, and reinforcing positive activities among peers.

As noted, your other efforts include raising parents' awareness about talking to their children about drugs and alcohol and giving them strategies for increasing their supervision. Additionally, you want parents to be aware of your efforts to provide alternative activities for youth and to reverse the "norm" around substance use. You decide to use many of the activities and tips from the public health campaign around "talking to your kids" (e.g., http://underagedrinking.samhsa.gov/talk-early.aspx) and to put these in the school newsletter that goes home to parents and on the Web sites of the elementary, middle, and high schools. Through your work with community leaders, the local police will increase surveillance around school events to ticket minors in possession of substances and provide increased screening of local convenience stores to ensure that tobacco and alcohol are not being sold to minors.

Now that you have the basics of your approach and your programming, you can begin to complete your logic model. Your resources or Inputs will include LifeSkills Training, after school programming, communication campaign with parents, and increased surveillance/enforcement from local authorities. Additionally, you'll have individuals who provide the

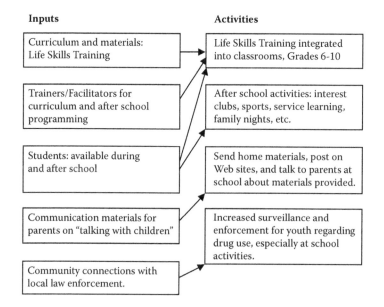

Figure 6.2   Preliminary steps of a program logic model.

LifeSkills Training and coordinate the after school activities as well as the participants (the students). You decide to focus your efforts on the two main activities: LifeSkills Training and the after school programming efforts. A preliminary program logic model is presented in Figure 6.2. It is read in the following manner: "If we have the following resources, we can provide the following activities."

CONCLUSION

Prior to developing and implementing a successful prevention or intervention plan, you must have a solid understanding of the issue of concern and the factors that contribute to its manifestation in your specific site. By using a combination of local data, research literature, and information from screening assessments, you should be able to develop a good understanding of the risk factors and protective factors that are contributing to the issue or concern in your setting. This information will help you to develop a comprehensive plan to address these factors at multiple levels. As you proceed with program planning, a solid logic model helps you to select and evaluate the critical elements of your plan.

Seven

Ecological Plan Implementation

Once your coalition has a clear understanding of the issue, the next step is to develop a plan. Hoefer (2006) describes this step as "deciding how to get from here to there" (p. 76). Use your preliminary logic model, described in Chapter 6, to guide the steps in your process. (See CD 7.1.) By mapping out the steps that will allow your coalition to reach its short- and long-term goals, you create a roadmap for your work.

INTERVENTION MAPPING

This is the stage of planning at which you are finalizing your logic model. Through your coalition building and data collection you have defined the unique *environmental elements and context* in which your interventions will occur. You are reviewing your *inputs*, stipulating the specific *activities* in which you will engage, and the *outputs* that you expect from those activities. From that, you have hypothesized which students will benefit and in which ways in the *short term*, *medium term*, and *long term*.

Determining Levels of Service

As outlined in Chapter 2, prevention services can be provided at different levels to meet the greatest number of student needs. When you are deciding on a plan, one of the decisions your team will need to make is the level(s) of prevention programming that is most appropriate for your unique concern and setting. Whether you decide at this time to provide services to all levels of need or not, best practice is to have considered all members of the population and their needs and to have made thoughtful decisions about what to provide for whom.

In making that decision, you'll want to consider both the prevalence and incidence within your setting. Prevalence refers to how often something occurs or how widespread it is. Sugai, Sprague, Horner, and Walker (2000) provided a general guideline that if 40% or more of your school is experiencing the identified concern or condition, then a universal intervention is warranted. Conversely, if less than 5% of your school population is at risk, then an indicated or selected level of prevention activity may be more appropriate. At times, the prevalence may not be great, but occurrences may be increasing and your team may decide to tackle the issue prior to it becoming widespread. Rising incidence rates suggests that greater primary prevention may be indicated. The severity and costliness of consequences of the specific concern may also drive the reasoning as to why it was selected as the target problem. Finally, a consideration of available resources is important to deciding the level of prevention that can be provided. Unfortunately, school systems often have to make difficult choices based on resource limitations. A clear understanding of how many students and to what severity they are being affected by a problem will help guide those difficult choices (and can be grounds for advocating for more resources).

Stipulating Temporal Frames

Depending on the issue that has been identified and the level of prevention, your team will want to establish timelines. As you evaluate your logic model, a consideration of when students become most at risk for a specific concern can be helpful in determining at which levels to target your prevention efforts. For example, we have evidence to suggest that students begin to disengage from school as early as third grade (O'Farrell, Morrison, & Furlong, 2006). If we wanted to develop a universal prevention program for school dropout, we would want to time our efforts to occur before or around the time that these initial signs of disengagement (e.g., decreased academic achievement, higher levels of absences, increased levels of acting out behaviors) are beginning to occur.

As a final temporal element, you'll want to consider the order of implementation. Which aspects of the plan have to be set in place before the next components can be added? This also will define the expected *outputs*. Given your implementation sequence, what duration, intensity, and frequency of what experience or intervention are you expecting which students to receive?

Evidence-Based Practices

Whether we're providing prevention or intervention, our programs must be based on the most sound research evidence. Additionally, prevention efforts can be broad and diffusely provided by individuals who do not have specific training in delivering programs (e.g., teachers, paraprofessionals). Therefore, the plan you select should have clear guidelines or a manual to increase the likelihood that it is implemented as planned.

In addition to the challenge of providing services to the greatest number of students, we must also ensure that those services we provide are likely to have the desired outcome. All aspects of our services, from prevention to intervention should reflect processes (e.g., assessment, identification, intervention) that are supported by research. The term *evidence-based practice* refers to programs or interventions that are not only based on sound scientific knowledge but also have been demonstrated to be effective through rigorous research (Hoagwood, Burns, & Weisz, 2002). By indicating that an approach is an evidence-based practice, we are saying that it has robust, empirical evidence to support its use with a particular issue or population. Unfortunately, there are many gaps in our knowledge about what works with which population and in what setting.

Although current research is beginning to address some of the problems with applying evidence-based practices in the schools, in the past there has been skepticism on the part of practitioners because many intervention studies were carried out in carefully controlled, clinical settings. The ability to adapt these approaches to "real world" settings seemed like a remote possibility at best because of the levels of comorbidity, the dynamic nature of schools, and the limited resources (e.g., time, expertise) available to deliver these interventions. Sadly, schools tend to adopt programs that have robust marketing campaigns and that are similar to other programs that have been used in the past. School personnel do not tend to select programs based on evidence of having been appropriately evaluated or that have been shown to produce the desired outcomes (Ennett et al., 2003). The end result has been that it is difficult to integrate evidence-based practices into public health settings, such as schools (Hoagwood & Johnson, 2003). In fact, Zins, Weissberg, Wang, and Walberg (2004) reported that although a typical school will deliver an average of 14 separate programs that address social–emotional issues, most will not be evidence based. Further, these programs often are not provided in a systematic manner.

Fortunately, school psychologists no longer have to conduct extensive library searches to find evidence-based programming. Various federal agencies, research centers, and private organizations have undertaken systematic reviews of available programs and created databases that list the numerous programs and their evidence, and provide guidance to consumers on how to select the best program for a specific need. For example, one of the educationally focused databases, the What Works Clearinghouse (http://ies.ed.gov/ncee/wwc/) established by the U.S. Department of Education, provides a centralized location for information on academic intervention programs and practices. Although the majority of the information on this site focuses on academic interventions, reports related to school completion and behavioral interventions for elementary school children have recently been added. Another excellent centralized source for evidence-based school-based mental health programming can be found at http://rtckids.fmhi.usf.edu/rtcpubs/study04/default.cfm. This guide, *School-Based Mental Health: An Empirical Guide for Decision-Makers,* a compilation of information from seven other databases (e.g., SAMHSA, Department of Education, Collaborative for Academic, Social, and Emotional Learning), lists a number of empirically supported school mental health programs designed to address a variety of different issues (e.g., substance abuse, acting out behavior) across different tiers of service and provides program information as well as estimated price per student.

As training programs, professional organizations, and professional literature continue to focus on evidence-based practices, it is likely that we will begin to see a shift toward more of this type of programming integrated into educational settings. However, Hoagwood and Johnson (2003) also concluded that "implementation and dissemination of EBPs [evidence-based practices] into service settings are likely to require a two-way adaptation: an adaptation of research design and methods to accommodate practice-related exigencies and an accommodation of practice settings to allow incorporation of EBPs" (p. 9). Additionally, we will need to gather a great deal more information on aspects of services beyond just intervention. As noted earlier, evidence-based practice is not reserved for interventions only; it applies also to screening, assessment, treatment, and all aspects of psychological services. Unfortunately, most of the work to date on evidence-based practices has focused exclusively on interventions and less so on identification and assessment procedures. To provide early intervention, we need reliable and valid methods for identifying those students who may have mental, emotional, or behavioral disorders.

Implementation Fidelity

As stated, we want to select an evidence-based intervention that contains enough specificity that it may be implemented with fidelity by various caregivers. It is critically important that the fidelity with which the interventions are implemented is assessed. A first step to evaluating the fidelity is to know what provision of the intervention constitutes, and conversely, what does not constitute provision of the intervention. In other words, does everyone on the team know what "is" and what "isn't" the intervention? Behavioral theory states that all behavior has three elements: frequency, intensity, and duration (Miltenberger, 2008). Operationalizing each intervention by these dimensions is a good starting place. A more sophisticated method of defining an intervention is Intervention Configuration Mapping (Hall & Hord, 2011). In a nutshell, each component of an intervention is defined, with all the various ways that it could be implemented. Then, through use and discussion of use, these descriptions are refined. The final step is to agree what variations exemplify the ideal implementation of the intervention, which variations are acceptable implementations, and which variations are unacceptable (or, are not the intervention). Ideally, you will be able to report to what degree of fidelity for which groups of students each intervention was provided.

COMMUNICATION AND EDUCATION
IN PLAN IMPLEMENTATION

In addition to making vital decisions about the who, when, and how of your plan, you also must develop clear lines of communication about the plan itself. Not everyone has been involved in the planning process, so to inform others about the proposed plan, you must engage in the process of informing your stakeholders (e.g., teachers, families, students, and community members) about aspects of the plan. Along with information sharing, there might be an educational component to your plan as well. To build the capacity described in Chapter 3, you will want to train people who can make a difference in the lives of children. Not only does this help to expand the reach of your program, but it also creates the potential for a greater degree of fidelity in implementation.

Providing Information

One of the first tasks of building capacity to enact positive change in your system is to educate your audience. As Kirkwood and Stamm (2006) aptly noted, "Change is voluntary and results from exposure to a properly positioned persuasive message" (p. 475). In other words, if you want to help others see the importance of engaging in different practices related to a targeted concern, you may have to work to help potential stakeholders see the value of such efforts. To apply this idea to a contemporary issue, consider the problem of school dropout. Some districts have experienced extremely high rates of school dropout and although concern was duly noted, few broad, systemic efforts were developed to reduce this problem. Too often, schools and communities were reluctant to act because they did not view the targeted issue as a problem (e.g., good riddance to difficult students), much less one for which valuable resources should be used. Although this situation has improved a bit with the advent of the No Child Left Behind Act (Pub. L. No. 107-110), which requires schools to track their graduation rates using a common formula, this issue has not been given the same attention as efforts related to building literacy or addressing the achievement gap. To build a coalition of stakeholders who are interested in tackling a targeted issue in your district, it is likely that you'll need to engage in *social marketing*. Kotler and Roberto (1989) define social marketing as organized efforts by one group (e.g., change agent) to persuade another group (e.g., target group) to accept or modify certain ideas, attitudes, and/or practices in lieu of others, preferably those that support the prevention efforts toward the targeted issue.

The public education framework promoted by Kirkwood and Stamm (2006) entails three broad steps: establish the audience and the message, develop and launch the campaign, and evaluate the campaign. If this sounds a bit overwhelming and beyond the scope of practice for school psychology, consider the ways you might have already implemented a public education campaign. For example, you have become aware that more and more students are complaining about bullying and aggressive acts on the playground. You would like to encourage the school leadership to adopt the Second Step curriculum (Committee for Children, 2010) because you are aware of the literature that suggests it is effective in decreasing conflicts on the playground. However, you are also aware that teachers are feeling overwhelmed with all they are expected to do and that they believe there are only a few "bad apples" who should be punished. You decide to bring your idea to the Building Leadership Team, the Student Wellness Team, or whichever entity in your school is responsible for making these kinds of decisions. You present your evidence of increased bullying and playground discipline referrals, you discuss the Second Step program and data related to its use in schools, and you present the logistics of implementing this program (e.g., purchase price, time, and training requirements). Based on your presentation, the team decides that more attention should be directed toward playground issues. They agree to collect additional data and explore various programs that are directed toward reducing playground problems. Although the team was hesitant to adopt a specific curriculum at this time, you believe you were successful as they are willing to look at this issue in more depth. If this scenario sounds familiar, you have engaged in public education and social marketing on a smaller scale.

Depending on the targeted issue and the breadth of its impact on the community, you may want to work in a broader context. Engaging parent groups, community agencies, and/or the targeted population and their families are all effective and necessary methods for assisting you in planning and implementing broad-based preventive programming. As another example, you may have identified increased gang activity, a larger number of adolescents experimenting with more dangerous substances (e.g., meth), or a higher than normal pregnancy rate among adolescents. Clearly these issues cannot be addressed by one individual, or even one organization. However, working together, various groups who are interested in the targeted issue can help identify the audience and the message that you want to deliver to those who are in a position to help create change. Additionally, using this group approach, especially if it includes the voice of those who are impacted by the issue (e.g., students who live in gang-infested neighborhoods), your work group can develop a deeper understanding of the issue and the ability to dialogue can lead to social action (Kirkwood & Stamm, 2006).

Once you've decided on your audience and your message, it is time to launch your "campaign," or your message. It is important that whatever format you use to raise public awareness, you stick to your evidence and adapt your message to fit your audience. You would not want to deliver a presentation full of technical jargon to a neighborhood parent group any more than you would want to deliver an impassioned plea to a funding agency. Your message should be simple and attractive, and you should be sure that you are getting the message out as broadly as possible. Consider multiple avenues for delivering your message, for example, newsletters, Web sites, flyers in community gathering places, displays, presentations, even radio air time (e.g., offer to be interviewed for a local interest show). Finally, your work group will need to evaluate your public education plan. (See CD 7.2.) How will you know that you have raised the awareness of the local community?

Although we'll address program evaluation in more depth in the next chapter, it is important from the beginning of your project to consider how you will evaluate all aspects of your process. Using the goal of reducing teen pregnancy as an example, let's say that you work with your group to develop a great plan, you have an energetic team on board, and when it comes time to deliver the intervention, you realize that you don't have enough participants or, worse yet, because of miscommunication, there is parent protest to your planned efforts. Your methods for monitoring the degree to which your communication is reaching the intended audience can be formal or informal (e.g., phone survey). You want to be sure that your message is reaching a good percentage of your intended audience and that the message that you're sending is being interpreted in the correct manner. One of the ways to avoid this type of problem is to be sure that you have developed a solid coalition of school staff, family members, and community representatives. These stakeholders can provide input, assistance, and decision-making at each step of your plan implementation.

Training of Caregivers and Service Providers

Facilitating a shared vision in school environments. School systems are hierarchical bureaucracies that can be resistant to change. Our Public Health Problem-Solving Model assumes shared power and responsibility in change. This can be threatening to the existing power structure. To facilitate a shared power model, it is important that all members of the system feel empowered.

Maton (2008) states that a shared vision is critical to establishing an empowering environment: A shared vision "encompasses a view of setting members [partners], including their needs and potential, and how they can work within the setting to achieve personal and setting goals" (p. 8). A shared vision should not be confused with a shared framework. Frameworks and assumptions are based on the individual's life experiences, societal roles, and worldview; given the different experiences of a diverse group, it cannot be assumed that the group will arrive at common frameworks and assumptions. Instead a realistic goal is a comprehensive group belief system that is based on a shared vision and includes the strategies for actualizing that vision. An understanding of each other's assumptions (and how they differ) maintains the commitment to the shared goals and allows each party to hold one another accountable when the inevitable problems and disagreements surface. See also Chapter 3 regarding coalition building.

Caregiver training and professional development: Considerations and logistics. To facilitate systemic change and increase the likelihood that your plan will be implemented with fidelity, training caregivers, services providers, and those individuals who can make a difference is a necessary component. Parents, classroom teachers, and community members (e.g., religious leaders, after school program leaders, athletic coaches) represent significant influences in a child's life. Mental health professionals can share their expertise with these individuals to help them more effectively communicate with children, create healthy environments, and identify children who are in need of additional mental health services.

One of the key features of caregiver training and professional development is to provide these training opportunities in context. Once you have established an interest group and have a core group of stakeholders, your group can begin the process of planning and deciding what types of training might be delivered, who should receive it, through what methods, and many other types of decisions related to this component.

The very act of training another individual suggests a power differential. You possess information or expertise that you are going to share with another. When your group is planning for training opportunities, it is important to be aware of this type of implied hierarchical relationship. For example, you wouldn't want to invite a group of parents to assist in planning an intervention to reduce student aggression and then allocate many of the meetings to parent training. The implied message might be that the school team views parents as the "problem" and they alone possess the knowledge and skills to "fix the problem." The same is true for ongoing professional development provided to teachers and paraprofessionals. In collaborative consultation, the expertise that each member of the team brings to the consultation process is recognized; similarly, making each participant's expertise and critical role explicit is important to support the empowerment and shared vision necessary to sustain the work.

Consider strategies for reducing the "top-down" provision of training through careful planning around when and where trainings will be held (e.g., day care centers, after school programs, YMCA/YWCA, community centers) and what types of services will be provided to facilitate participation (e.g., child care, transportation). Your goal is to maximize family and community access and to encourage other members to organize and host meetings and trainings. Additionally, consider trainings that are delivered to the entire collaborative group and provided by an outside party. Are there parent or community groups who can provide training or professional development to school staff to help them better understand a cultural or mental health issue from another perspective? When school members provide training to the collaborative group, ensure that the topic area is one that is considered critical for achieving the collective goals of the entire group.

If you have created a broad, diverse group of stakeholders, members of this group who represent family or community members can help identify additional individuals to involve. For example, they can help identify and share information with family members who might be interested in receiving the training, or they may know of community members who are knowledgeable about particular topics. By networking with a larger group, it is more likely that you'll be able to find presenters, consultants, and additional community members who share similarities in culture, ethnicity, race, language, and socioeconomics with your identified audience (Nelson, Prilleltensky, & MacGillivary, 2001). Broad input also allows your group to obtain information about the community so that you can adapt interventions as needed to address specific community-identified needs and goals.

Caregiver training and professional development: Content and presentation. The potential content areas for the trainings will vary based on the goals of your project, but they will likely include topics within a school psychologist's expertise, such as parenting, classroom and school discipline, behavior management, child development, or basic communication skills. If your group has selected a particular program, trainings might be provided by an outside organization such as the creators of the program or a local agency that has been using the approach. If partnering with a university, faculty members might provide training in evaluating your project or strategies for enhancing your collaboration (e.g., problem-solving, decision-making, policy development). Finally, there may be community agencies that can provide training such as strategies for working with members of a particular ethnic or cultural group, understanding how a particular system works (e.g., juvenile justice, mental health), or another perspective on the issue that your group plans to address (e.g., gang involve-ment from the perspective of former gang members). Trainings may be directed at improving the group's process (e.g., com-munication skills), enhancing the broader knowledge of the group to facilitate decision-making (e.g., culturally responsive practice with a specific group), and providing information such as how to implement the specific intervention (e.g., steps in implementing a program with fidelity).

From this perspective, training needs may also match the levels of prevention activities (e.g., universal, selective, indi-cated). That is, consider what preparation all stakeholders need to create an appropriate context for the implementation of a program. If you are working to implement whole school reform, what information or skills are needed to increase the chances that your efforts will be successful? For example, if your group decided that a school-wide PBIS approach would decrease the levels of aggression that you are seeing among students, there are certain steps that your group might take to prepare the school and community members for imple-mentation of such a program. Your group might provide data on reported levels of aggression and bullying, evidence of long-term negative effects of bullying, information on what a school-wide positive behavioral approach entails, as well as supportive data. The goals for this type of training are to help make others aware of the issue and the importance of taking action, and to help all school staff and families understand the program and the types of changes that would be required. Once the program is officially implemented in the school, the types of training might become a bit more focused by working with various grade-level teachers to adapt aspects of the pro-gramming to meet the developmental needs of their students or training with other school staff (e.g., bus driver, custodian, office administration, lunch room staff) to help them better understand how to implement aspects of the program within their own context. A framework for planning your education and advocacy efforts is provided on CD 7.3. At the most narrow level, you may have what could be considered "troubleshooting" to address the needs of individuals who are reluctant or struggling to implement the program or doing so in a manner that is contrary to your efforts.

CONCLUSION

Implementing a plan from the Public Health Problem-Solving Model is both a daunting and "do-able" opportunity. A key to the success of intervention implementation is to have a clear vision of the plan. A well-developed logic model is critical for establishing the sequence and expected outcomes of the plan. Within that logic model, you want to stipulate the levels of service that will be provided to which recipients, specify the sequence and timing of the interventions, ensure that the research supports your expected outcomes, and establish a means of measuring treatment integrity. Communication and education about the intervention is as important as the plan development for the successful outcomes of your project. This requires providing information to a broad constituency as well as training to those who will be implementing the interventions. As all interventions occur within a dynamic context, continual monitoring and plan refinements will be necessary.

Eight

Monitoring and Evaluating Outcomes

A n essential component of any sustained effort at systemic reform is a thorough evaluation that is carefully integrated into all aspects of the model. We must be accountable for our efforts and ensure that they are effective in supporting student achievement. Results evaluation is an emphasized component of *Blueprint III* (Ysseldyke et al., 2006) and the NASP Practice Model (NASP, 2010).

There are many reasons to conduct a program evaluation, but one of the most important is to determine whether your efforts are having the intended effects and whether this change is occurring to a meaningful degree. In your evaluation, you not only want to establish whether your efforts are effective but also whether they are being implemented with integrity, are accessible to the intended audience, have social validity, and are cost-effective (Power et al., 2003). Through these various approaches, collaborative groups can make informed decisions about which programs and efforts to continue and expand; those that hold promise, but may need some modification; and those that should be discontinued.

MEASURING PREVENTION IMPACTS

One of the difficulties of prevention research is that you are trying to establish that your group's efforts resulted in the absence of a negative outcome. For example, imagine that your team implemented a program that was designed to increase decision-making and problem-solving skills and decrease the incidence of teen pregnancy in a particular population. At the end of the program and at 1-year follow-up, you may be able to show that the young women who participated in your program improved in the targeted skills (i.e., decision-making, problem-solving) and might also find that the pregnancy rate

among participants was lower than in girls who did not participate. However, you are not able to say with absolute certainty
that the girls in your program would have become pregnant
and it was through participation in your program that they
did not. Those kind of definitive statements are not a part of
prevention research. Instead, we demonstrate how our results
align in the expected ways with our model of intervention.

Just as the logic model presented in Chapter 6 can be used to
guide your group in developing a program, it also provides the
framework for the evaluation of your program. In your model,
you have defined what you think will change based on your
program and, to some degree, why you think it will change (e.g.,
your theory of change). Program logic models are even more
detailed and will detail your *inputs* (e.g., planned activities,
resources) as well as your *outputs* and *outcomes* (Knowlton &
Phillips, 2009). The graphic nature of the logic model allows
your team to easily look at and plan for the evaluation of all of
the program components (e.g., *inputs, activities, outputs,* and
outcomes [short term, medium term, and long term]), as well as

the significant contextual and environmental variables of your
prevention or intervention programming. (See CD 8.1.)

EMPOWERMENT THROUGH
THE EVALUATION PROCESS

Involvement of important stakeholders does not end with the
selection and planning of prevention and program efforts.
Families, teachers, administrators, and community members
should be included in program evaluation efforts as well. If
individuals are involved at all stages of program development,
implementation, and evaluation, it is more likely that you will
have "buy in" and members will feel empowered as decision-
makers. This enhanced role of family members from research
respondents to research consultants allows families to have a
much greater influence on research agendas and marks a significant change from traditional program evaluation (Friesen
& Stephens, 1998). When programs focus on children and adolescents from diverse backgrounds, it is especially important
to encourage family and student inclusion (Roosa, Dumka,
Gonzales, & Knight, 2002).

Nastasi et al. (2000) described a participatory intervention
model that provides a framework for involving community
members, family members, and others in the planning and

evaluation of intervention efforts. The objectives of empowerment evaluation are to increase the probability of program
success through providing stakeholders with the tools to
assess the planning, implementation, and evaluation of their
program, and to mainstream evaluation activities within the
organization (Fetterman & Wandersman, 2005). Applied to
the Public Health Problem-Solving Model, this would mean
that one outcome we seek is that all participants and stakeholders are able to assess the outcomes of the interventions
and become more sophisticated evaluators of other services
as well, with the intent that this empowerment and increased
skill set will support successful student outcomes.

PROCESS EVALUATION: EVALUATION
OF PROGRAM IMPLEMENTATION

The first question to address is how your program was delivered and to whom. Power et al. (2003) described this step as
process evaluation and noted that it helps to establish whether
the program was delivered to the targeted group (e.g., entire
school, grade level, or students at risk for depression). Within a
logic model framework, this step would assess the *inputs* and
activities of the programming. These are measured through
the use of *process indicators*. The types of data collected at
this level might include information on the dates a program
was delivered, duration of the sessions as well as overall
length of program (e.g., 6 weeks), and who received the program on which dates. There are many important reasons to
consider these variables, especially in school settings where
school breaks, student and staff absences, and scheduling difficulties can all affect program delivery.

Consider an example where your Building Leadership Team
decides to implement a targeted prevention program (e.g.,
Second Step) across the third- and fourth-grade class levels
to address increased levels of bullying behaviors on the playground. Your team decides to evaluate whether the program
is having the desired effect (e.g., reduced number of office
referrals generated during recess times) after 8 weeks of implementation. Unfortunately, you find there has been no change;
office referrals occurring during recess periods remain the
same as they were prior to the implementation of the program.
Your group might conclude that the program simply needs
more time to be effective or that it does not work for your

population. In either case, your conclusions might not be correct without further exploration.

Instead, your team then decides to approach the teachers to gather information about program implementation. You find that due to state-mandated testing and spring break, the program was not delivered 3 of the 8 weeks and that the sessions had been shortened to 15 to 20 minutes in two of the classrooms. At this point, your team is better prepared to make decisions about next steps. First, you would want to have discussions around when to implement (e.g., at a different time of day, at a different point in the year), whether staff need more training in program implementation or more program "buy in," or whether this program is the best choice given the limitations of the setting. Process indicators are very important to consider before determining whether a program has resulted in the intended outcome.

An equally important question related to program delivery is the quality of implementation. Power et al. (2003) describe this program evaluation component as "integrity." The question of integrity is much more complicated and difficult to determine. There are also a number of different methods to gather this information, but some of them are costly in terms of time and resources. For example, direct observation is a common method for determining the quality of program implementation. This strategy requires that there is some rubric or template for the various program components, and the observer measures the observed implementation to this standard. This method is most effective when there is a standardized method of delivery. If the implementation is not designed to be delivered in a highly structured format, the question of quality implementation is subject to "the eye of the beholder." However, if there is a manualized script that is to be delivered as part of the program, then it is much more likely that any individual observing that session would draw similar conclusions regarding the quality of implementation. Using the earlier example of implementing Second Steps in several classrooms, it means that observers would need to go into each of those classrooms at different points through program implementation to observe for fidelity of implementation.

Broadly defined, program fidelity refers to the degree to which a program was delivered as designed. Power et al. (2003) provided a specific definition as the "percentage of program steps that were provided correctly" (p. 195). Clearly, it would be difficult to have observers go to all of those sessions on a regular basis, and it is also possible that program delivery might vary based on whether a session is being observed or not. Another alternative described by Power et al. is a self-report of implementation integrity. Using this approach, after each session, the teacher or whoever was delivering the intervention would check the steps or components of the program that were delivered according to a specific template that lists program steps (much like the form that might be used by an observer).

This method of integrity checking also has drawbacks in that self-report checklists are subject to bias (Power et al., 2003). Another alternative for assessing program integrity is assessing products generated from the project. For, example, videotapes of sessions could be reviewed and rated to determine the degree to which program steps were implemented. If all sessions were taped and only random sessions were selected for viewing, it might help to ensure a higher quality of program delivery overall (Power et al., 2003). When possible, all three strategies would be used to ensure the quality of program delivery. This information can be used to provide both positive and constructive feedback to those delivering the programming and to make decisions as to whether additional training is needed.

Each of these methods is focused on the content of the program and may overlook other aspects of quality. For example, when considering a manualized treatment delivered in a therapeutic setting, the therapist might deliver the intervention exactly as specified in the manual. However, if the relationship between client and therapist is not present, it is unlikely that the intervention will be efficacious. Depending on the type of program and the likelihood that these more qualitative aspects might affect outcomes, it is also important to determine methods of assessing these components as well. In addition to observing content components of the program, observers could take note of various indicators of relationship between the program provider and the audience. Another method for collecting data on the relationship might include interviews with the program participants and their families (Power et al., 2003).

One final aspect of your process evaluation is to consider the degree to which you have communicated your efforts with others. Are you attracting attention to your issue? Have you raised awareness? Are your stakeholders and your audiences moved by your message? These are the types of evaluative questions you might ask. These types of questions help you to evaluate your advocacy efforts (discussed in Chapter 11).

OUTCOME EVALUATION: EVALUATING IMPACTS OF A PROGRAM

After measuring indicators related to the process and integrity of a program, it is appropriate to measure outcomes. From your logic model, you will monitor both the targeted condition as well as the risk or protective factors associated with your theory of change. For example, let's assume your team has decided to implement the Incredible Years program in four preschools located in your district. Your team has read the research suggesting it is an effective program at reducing aggression because it helps families improve their child management skills and it helps young children to increase their self-regulation. Your logic model would be represented in this manner (see Figure 8.1). Basically, it states that when parents have improved child management skills and children are directly taught strategies for improving their self-regulation, previously aggressive children will be better able to manage their feelings of frustration and anger. Further, through consistent, firm parenting, children will learn more appropriate actions in response to these negative feelings. As parents and children increase in both of these skills, children will show reductions in aggressive behaviors and, in the long term, have more positive adaptive and social outcomes.

Although not reflected in this model, the reason for selecting child management skills and self-regulation as the targeted areas for intervention reflects our knowledge of the condition (i.e., higher rates of aggressive behaviors in preschool populations). Research has indicated that parents who have poor discipline skills (risk factor) and children with poor ability to regulate their emotions (risk factor) are more at risk for aggressive behaviors and negative long-term outcomes.

In monitoring our outcomes, we will examine changes in the incidence and prevalence of the targeted condition (i.e., aggressive behaviors) as well as changes in risk factors (parenting behavior and self-regulation). As indicated in the model represented in Figure 8.1, *outcome indicators* may include short- and long-term outcomes. It is important to keep in mind that there are a lot of potential indicators that you could use to measure whether your program was effective. Power et al.

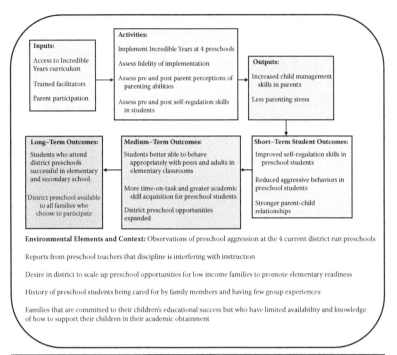

Figure 8.1 Logic model for addressing preschool aggression.

(2003) advocate that outcomes are measured in terms of the effectiveness of the program as well as the social validity of the intervention for the program participants. Because children's behavior often varies from one situation to the next, you may want to evaluate outcomes across settings (McConaughy & Leone, 2002). However, you also don't want to select so many indicators that it is almost impossible to obtain and track all of your data. Instead, it is important to pick a few key indicators that are relatively easy to track. The following questions can help your team decide which ones to monitor (Horsch, 1997):

- Is the indicator relevant—does it enable you to know about the expected result or condition?
- Is the indicator defined and data collected in the same way over time?
- Will data be available for the indicator?
- Are data for the indicator currently being collected or can cost-effective instruments for data collection be developed?
- Will the indicator provide sufficient information about a condition or result to convince both supporters and skeptics?
- Is the indicator quantifiable?

In prevention programming, we're typically working to reduce risk as well as promote protective factors. As a result, we should ensure that the outcomes that we are monitoring include both of these components (McConaughy & Leone, 2002). For example, in addition to determining whether playground disciplinary referrals have decreased in number, we would also want to evaluate whether problem-solving behaviors increased through playground observations and/or self-report indices. It is important that we select methods that are both reliable and valid, as well as those that measure the targeted construct as closely as possible (McConaughy & Leone, 2002). Using your logic model, you would expect to see decreases in certain behaviors over the short term, such as fewer playground disciplinary referrals. Conversely, you might also expect to see an increase in the self-reported use of problem-solving strategies. Student self-reports would be supported by direct observations of problem-solving behaviors in the classroom using a rating scale designed for playground observations. In other words, you would expect the variables to change in accordance with your logic model.

In addition to short-term indicators, you would also want to look at medium- and long-term outcomes. If your program was effective in reducing bullying behavior on the playground, a school climate indicator at the end of the year might reflect that students rate themselves as feeling safer at school and rules as being enforced more consistently than they rated these same things at the beginning of the year (medium-term outcomes). Obviously, assessing the change across the year necessitates collecting data prior to starting the program. Although we have not discussed program evaluation until now, good program evaluations are designed concurrent to the development of the programs they evaluate, and each helps to strengthen the other; in other words, establishing how you want to evaluate outcomes should improve the program delivery design, and a well-thought-out program will make it clear what outcomes should be evaluated and how that will occur.

Although sense of safety and consistent rule enforcement are not direct measures of a program that targeted bullying behaviors, it would be expected that these might be long-term outcomes that would result if there were fewer bullying incidents. In the Power et al. (2003) model, this type of indicator would reflect the "social validity" of the program. At this level, the question is asked, "What value did the program have for the community?" (Power et al., 2003, p. 199). In order for a program to be sustained over time, it needs to be viewed as valuable and acceptable to the community. If the program doesn't appear to make a "real" change in significant aspects of functioning, stakeholders will tend to look for other programs that have a greater impact, or they may simply reduce their involvement in the current efforts.

EFFECTIVENESS AND EFFICACY RESEARCH

Once your team has measured impact on the incidence and prevalence of the targeted conditions as well as other outcomes (intended and unintended), a more advanced step is to analyze if your outcomes are real, or simply fluctuations in human behavior. This task involves knowledge of descriptive and inferential statistical models that will allow you to estimate the significance and contributors to the observed changes. A further step is also to consider the most efficient means (financially and expediently) to accomplish these outcomes. This level of analysis is beyond the scope of this book and beyond the means of most building-level practitioners. Some larger districts have in-house research departments that can assist in these activities; also, there are external evaluation companies that provide evaluation services for a fee, as well as university partners that can assist in these evaluations.

CONCLUSION

Although evaluation is listed as the last stage of the Public Health Problem-Solving Model, your program evaluation will be most successful if it is considered to be an integral aspect of all program planning. Measuring the impact of prevention is particularly tricky and not completely possible. For this reason, it is critically important that your logic model stipulates the expected outcomes for particular groups of students so that inferences can be drawn. Partnering with constituents on the evaluation makes the evaluation process an opportunity to empower the community with which you are working. Program evaluation consists of consideration of the implementation of the program and examination of the outcomes.

III

FROM CONCEPT TO ACTION

The evil that is in the world almost always comes of ignorance, and good intentions may do as much harm as malevolence if they lack understanding.

—**Albert Camus**

As the opening quote illustrates, without understanding of the local conditions as well as our possible role in these conditions, we can perpetuate or exacerbate that which we seek to challenge. Therefore, this section is designed to provide support so that you may confidently establish your Public Health Problem-Solving Model of practice that does indeed support comprehensive mental health services for all students.

Chapter 9 walks you through the stages of the Public Health Problem-Solving Model as applied to a case study in one elementary school. Key steps are outlined for each stage. This case study makes apparent that it takes a team of dedicated individuals to create meaningful, comprehensive change.

In Chapter 10, we tackle the changes to the role of school psychologist that will be required if you are to practice the Public Health Problem-Solving Model. We provide parallels between the skills that all school psychologists are expected to develop and the necessary skills for a school psychologist practicing from the Public Health Problem-Solving Model. We also provide techniques for avoiding burnout as you take on this challenging and critical work.

The final chapter of the book, Chapter 11, discusses how to sustain the changes that are possible through the Public Health Problem-Solving Model. Without attention to maintaining system change, the improvements that were realized may not become institutionalized. Monitoring, advocacy, persuasion, and negotiation are important activities in maintaining change. When viewed through a social justice lens, this model provides a framework for achieving the equity and access to services that is fundamental to the long-standing goals of school psychologists.

Nine

Case Study in Public Health Problem-Solving

ANSEL ADAMS ELEMENTARY SCHOOL

Ansel Adams Elementary School is a fairly large elementary school located in a suburban community of about 90,000 people. The community itself is somewhat segregated with most of the Latino population and those with lower incomes living in the north, east, and southern-most areas of town, while the western half of the community is populated predominantly with White, non-Latino families from the middle to upper socioeconomic strata. Ansel Adams Elementary is located in the very northeast corner of the city. As a result, the majority of the students are eligible for free lunch or reduced lunch (>85%), most of the students are Latino (95%), and a majority of these students are considered to be English-language learners (~65%). The surrounding neighborhood around the school is considered to be dangerous. Many individuals are out of work and spend their afternoons on the porches of their houses gathering with their friends and drinking. The dropout rate is high, and many adolescents are also out on the streets; too many have become involved in selling and using drugs. Because many of the families are not in the country legally, those who are employed work difficult jobs with long hours; these factors limit their ability to connect with the school.

With the recent economic downturn, problems in the community and school have gone from bad to worse. Many children are deeply affected by the loss of income in their households. Families are living together, some are now homeless and living in shelters, and the general level of stress has gone up in nearly every home. At school, the students seem distracted, distressed, and are engaging in more fights, both verbal and physical, with their peers. Recognizing that the issue reflects a broader community problem, the school psychologist and school counselor decide to work together to develop a plan to address the problem. They first approach their principal, who is a strong leader but relatively new to that school. The principal agrees that this is an important issue and gives them the go-ahead. They also enlist the help of a couple of the members of the school's small but devoted group of parent volunteers to participate in their program planning. A template for a sample invitation letter is provided on the CD (9.1).

KEY STEPS IN GETTING STARTED

- Recognize the need for a different kind of approach.
- Get permission from administration to form a group of stakeholders to address the broad issue of concern.
- Begin inviting members from the school, families, and community organizations to join an interest group.
    - Invite your initial members through personal invitations. Subsequent invitations may be made either personally or through letters to potential members.
    - Your initial gathering may be small. Have group members identify other potential group members.
    - Begin to establish your process (e.g., when and how often you will meet, where you will meet, how long the meetings will last, how the meetings will be organized).
    - Consider writing a small internal grant to obtain funding to provide snacks and child care at meetings.

STAGE 1: PROBLEM IDENTIFICATION THROUGH APPLIED EPIDEMIOLOGY

Together, you (the school psychologist), the school counselor, parent volunteers, and community members build a plan. You first want to understand more about what is happening in the classroom, on the playgrounds, and at home. You develop a list of people to interview and a common set of questions so that the group can gather some preliminary information to help explain the behaviors they are seeing at school. Because you have bilingual parent volunteers on the team, they are able to identify some Spanish-speaking families to interview. These volunteers also suggest interviewing some community leaders (e.g., a priest at a local church, director of the community recreation center) to gather their insights.

When all of this information is brought back to a subsequent group meeting, a measurable set of concerns is identified, and the group agrees that these will be their areas of focus. The people interviewed describe both internalizing type issues associated with anxiety (e.g., crying easily, worry, difficulty sleeping) as well as externalizing problems (e.g., aggressive behaviors such as hitting, pushing, threats, and name-calling). Some of the identified behavioral concerns appear to be directly related to lack of resources (e.g., poor hygiene, hunger, lack of sleep, and related learning problems associated with these conditions such as difficulty concentrating). Although the reports of this behavior are minimal, some teachers report seeing a greater level of stealing within their classrooms.

As part of the first step in identifying and operationalizing clear and measurable targets for intervention, school personnel (e.g., school psychologist, school counselor, principal, teachers) collaborate with parents to develop the criterion of four or more behaviors (both internalizing and externalizing) as areas of concern. After developing a standard list of concerning behaviors, teachers are asked to report the number of students in their class who exhibited four or more of the behaviors in the last month. In the school population of 640 students, teachers report a total of 115 students with a concerning behavior score of 4 or more. Using the formula presented in Chapter 4, it is determined that the school prevalence rate for concerning behaviors (as defined by the stakeholders) is about 18% (115/640 × 100). At this point, no specific students have been identified, and the information has only been used to establish a prevalence rate. This information provides an indication to the working group (i.e., school psychologist, school counselor, principal, and parent and community members) of the degree of the problem.

KEY STEPS IN PROBLEM IDENTIFICATION

- Gather preliminary data through interviews, observations, and screening measures.
- Define specific areas of concern and establish prevalence.
- Establish which groups of students may be experiencing the greatest levels of risk.

STAGE 2: PROBLEM ANALYSIS OF RISK FACTORS AND PROTECTIVE FACTORS

Your working group then begins to gather information about the potential risk factors and protective factors associated with some of the concerning behaviors that they are seeing. Through a brief literature review, background experience, and parental input, your working group is able to identify a number of potential risk and protective factors associated with concerning behaviors identified at Ansel Adams Elementary School.

Clearly, community factors are placing these students at risk (e.g., dangerous neighborhoods, lack of resources, isolation), but also there are risks at the family, school, peer, and individual levels. At the family level, some of the identified risk factors include mental health concerns (e.g., depression), substance abuse, and unemployment. At school, the inconsistent application of rules, low teacher expectations, and high rates of teacher turnover and non-licensed teachers may be contributing to the concerns. A number of these risk and protective factors are associated with characteristics of the students themselves (e.g., previous history of trauma, poor coping skills, lack of friends) as well as of their peers (e.g., deviant peers).

Some of the identified protective factors across these five contexts include key community agencies and churches that have strong connections to some of the families in the school's catchment area, a core group of family volunteers who are willing to assist, and strong leadership within the school building. The working group develops an operationalized list of the potential risk and protective factors that are most closely associated with the concerning behaviors observed at Ansel Adams, along with ways to measure each factor. Through surveys of students, parents, and school personnel, the working group is able to gather some information but they also gather data from the school's database (e.g., attendance, grades, achievement scores, discipline records). The group gathers more information on the community, district, and school to better understand the problems faced by families and resources that are available to them. Your working group analyzes all of the information and presents it to the school staff as well as interested community members and parents. The goal of this step is to identify the degree to which each of the identified risk and protective factors is present in the school and the local community. Table 9.1 shows a summary of the risk and protective factors associated with each of the

Table 9.1   Risk and Protective Factors Table for __Internalizing and Externalizing Behaviors, Learning Problems, Poor Health Behaviors____(Issue)

Risk Factors	Domain	Protective Factors
Inhibited (internalizing) or disinhibited (externalizing) temperament Previous history of trauma Poor coping strategies Mental health concerns (e.g., depression, anxiety),	**Individual**	Able to accomplish age-appropriate tasks Problem-solving coping strategies
Substance abuse Inconsistent discipline Low SES and unemployment	**Family**	Warm, supportive parent or caregiver Positive family environment Adequate supervision & monitoring
Peer rejection Deviant peers	**Peers**	Social support Positive reciprocal friendships
Inconsistent discipline and rules High turnover rate among teachers, many are unlicensed Low expectations for student achievement	**School**	Safe school climate Supportive adult at school Parents involved in education and strong school leadership
Lack of resources Poor role models (e.g., high rates of unemployment and drug use) Unsafe neighborhood	**Community**	A few strong community agencies and churches

behaviors of concern. Because your team recognizes that many of these factors are interrelated, you decide not to break each of the risk and protective factors out by area of concern; you simply group all risk factors together across concerns and do this for all protective factors as well.

STAGE 3: DEFINE RISK IN CHILD– ENVIRONMENT INTERACTIONS

At this point, the working group has prevalence data on the concerning behaviors as well as a much better understanding of the various risk and protective factors that might be impacting the high rate of concerning behaviors. It is clear from the table that some of the risk and protective factors are not amenable to change (e.g., student intelligence, lack of resources in the community). However, there are some clues as to where

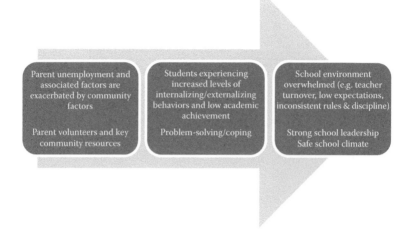

Figure 9.1   Risk and protective model for Ansel Adams Elementary School.

to begin. From this list of concerning behavioral problems and associated risk and protective factors, the working group collaborates with parents, students, administrators, teachers, and support personnel to develop a tentative causal model for current behavioral concerns evidenced at Ansel Adams Elementary School.

Figure 9.1 reflects the team's hypothesis about the sequence of events and interactions of the risk and protective variables that culminate in the behavioral concerns observed at Ansel Adams Elementary School. Although the arrow seems to reflect a linear process, there is a transactional component between student and school variables. That is, students may be experiencing more problems because supportive school environmental conditions are limited (e.g., high teacher turnover, inconsistent discipline) and the school environment is overwhelmed by the increasing needs of students. In this model, it is recognized that the problems became even worse after the change in the economy and parental employment levels. From the data gathered in the previous step, the working group develops a working risk/protection model. This model integrates existing research and theory on social and behavioral development of internalizing and externalizing problems with stakeholders' knowledge about specific characteristics of their setting.

The issues seem complicated as there are multiple behaviors of concern, but many are interconnected. For example, it is likely that both internalizing and externalizing behaviors are related to higher levels of stress and an increasingly disrupted school environment. Therefore, it may not be necessary to create a separate program to address each type of behavior. Additionally, your team might hypothesize that the higher levels of stress, aggression, and poor health (e.g., hunger, lack of sleep) are contributing to the falling grades. Therefore, if your intervention targets the poor coping, aggression, and health behaviors, you will see a resulting rise in academic performance. Based on this working model, your group begins to explore prevention programs that might help to decrease risk factors and strengthen protective factors associated with the school, family, peers, and students.

KEY STEPS IN PROBLEM ANALYSIS

- Identify and measure risk factors across settings (e.g., individual, family, peers, school, & community).
- Identify protective factors across settings.
- Create a model to explain the relationship between targeted concerns and the identified risk and protective factors.

Through a process of brainstorming, research, and knowledge of available resources in the district, your team begins to formulate a plan. Your team recognizes that there is no way to address every concern; therefore, they will need to make some decisions based on the number of students who are impacted, the type of resources that are available, and the nature of the concern. Generally speaking, the greater number of students who are experiencing the concern, the more likely your team will want to consider a universal approach. Before your team can implement your plans, you must consider two main components for your initiative:

1. Determining levels of service
2. Stipulating temporal frames

Determining levels of service. One of the first things your team needs to think about is the level at which they want to intervene. Because 18% of the students appear to be experiencing behaviors of concern, the team decides that a broad-based universal programming will likely result in the best outcomes.

Starting from the community level, the team decides to invite members from law enforcement to be on the planning committee. Through this connection, the team hopes to increase surveillance and enforcement around the school in the mornings and afternoons so that students are safer in their walk to and from school each day. The team recognizes that little can be done to increase parent employment; instead, they hope to reduce some of the strain of unemployment and lack of resources by connecting families to resources (e.g., food, assistance with rent, utilities, and clothing). Additionally, many families are not aware of the degree to which stress regarding money can affect children, and the team decides to provide information about how to talk appropriately to children about unemployment and money concerns.

At the school level, the most concerning factor is inconsistent discipline and rules. One of the reasons that many teachers are unhappy and overwhelmed is the degree of discipline problems at the school. It is believed that if these behavioral issues can be reduced, teachers will be less likely to leave the school and may begin to have higher expectations for student achievement. The district has a model for positive behavioral support, and there was a plan in place at Ansel Adams. However, with the rapid teacher turnover, many of the new teachers were not trained and the system is not being applied consistently. By reviving the Ansel Adams Positive Behavioral Interventions and Supports (PBIS) program and implementing teacher training for consistent application of school rules, some of the behavioral concerns will likely be reduced. Finally, students need strategies to cope with these life changes and the district happens to have the I Can Problem Solve (Shure & Spivak, 1988) curriculum available. The team will determine whether it is possible to implement this type of curriculum into the daily class routine.

Protective factors are also considered. For example, the parent volunteers are enlisted to help set up a resource fair to be held at the school. In conjunction with parent–teacher conferences, local community agencies and churches will be invited to set up tables that will have materials related to food and clothing banks, general equivalency diploma (GED) and English as a second language (ESL) classes, and utility/rental assistance, as well as low cost sources for family activities (e.g., public library) and support (e.g., pro bono mental health resources, support groups). As part of this fair, they will offer materials related to educating families about how to manage economic stress, talking to children about money, and keeping children safe.

The community agency members will also enlist volunteers within their own organizations. They decide to implement a food program that has been used in other communities where the food from various restaurants, stores, farmer's markets, and institutional cafeterias (e.g., universities, governmental agencies) is gathered and distributed. These items are provided to families in need, especially over weekends and holidays to help ensure that students have consistent access to food. The strong leadership in the school will help the team in obtaining teacher buy-in and implementation of the various plans. Because the team is working from a causal model, they also have their preliminary logic model as outlined in Chapter 6 (see Figure 9.2).

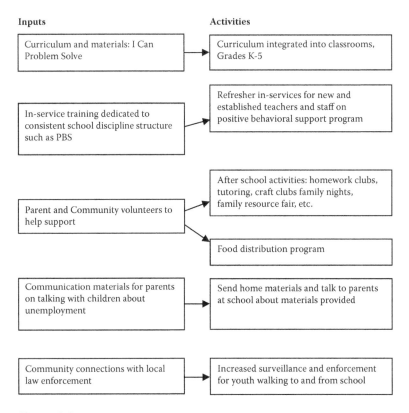

Figure 9.2   Preliminary logic model for Ansel Adams Elementary School.

As noted, the team prioritizes a universal approach early on in their planning. They want to start with a broad-based approach but also recognize that they need to reevaluate whether to also implement indicated and selective programming. If they are building programming at the more intensive levels into their plan, they can focus on specialized groups for students who have higher levels of risk (e.g., their families are homeless) or whose behaviors are indicating early signs of disorder (e.g., high levels of aggression, missing multiple days of school due to social anxiety). At the family level, they can create targeted parent education and support groups for those parents who are struggling the most.

Stipulating temporal frames. Sometimes primary prevention efforts can suffer from lack of clarity and direction because the activities are primarily implemented by nonprofessionals or professionals who are not trained in prevention and clinical work. Therefore, it is important to clearly define expectations, guidelines for implementation, timelines, and order of implementation for each of your efforts. At this point, the team divides into a few different working groups so that each can develop their implementation plan, which includes a clear definition of the interventions and their goals. In some instances, this plan might appear to be a bit looser (e.g., extra police patrols, food collection program). However, other components need to be much more defined, such as integration of the problem-solving curriculum into the school day. Your team has selected two evidence-based interventions (i.e., I Can Problem Solve and School-Wide Positive Behavioral Interventions and Supports) that should effectively address many of the behavioral concerns and overall adjustment. However, these programs must be delivered with fidelity in order to be effective. Therefore, the small task team needs to consider the logistics of delivering the program, such as when it will be taught each day, how teachers will be prepared to teach the curriculum, how implementation will be monitored, and other critical details. In some instances, aspects of a program may need to be developed. For example, creating an after school homework program is a good start, but there may be program elements that can make it even more effective.

Once these plans have been developed, the teams must consider order of implementation. Which aspects of the plan should be implemented first? Is there a logical order of implementation? Is there a timing issue (e.g., a holiday or testing window is approaching)? Is there a developmental variable such that students at the intermediate grades are more vulnerable than at the youngest grades? With your group, you decide that your top three priorities are safety (i.e., increased police surveillance in the mornings and afternoons), basic needs (i.e., food distribution program and resource fair), and behavior (i.e., revitalizing the school-wide PBIS program at Ansel Adams Elementary). The team decides to wait on implementation of the I Can Problem Solve program until later, at the beginning of the next semester.

STAGE 4: ECOLOGICAL PLAN IMPLEMENTATION

Your team is finally ready to implement the plans that have been developed. The first two steps are to provide information to the broader community and to provide professional development and training.

Providing information. Your team is finally ready to share their work with the broader school community, families of students in the school, and community members. You know how important it is to have buy-in from as many people as possible so that your plan will be implemented; thus your team works hard to create a campaign to inform others about the concerns, contributing factors, and the plan for improving conditions. As you are developing educational materials, your team considers how to reach as many family and community members as possible. Together, the team develops a multi-pronged approach. A meeting for all school personnel will occur during an upcoming teacher in-service day. A few different meetings will be held around town to help inform families about new programs that will be delivered at the school and new resources that are available. Additionally, some of the family volunteers agree to post information about the meetings in their places of work, on church bulletin boards, and through word of mouth. For parents who cannot attend, flyers will be sent that are written in English and Spanish.

If your team decides they need additional funding to enact the plan, members from your group may need to approach community members for funding. If so, your group will need to consider ways to deliver information quickly, concisely, and in a compelling manner such that potential funders respond favorably. The term *elevator speech* has been used in many different contexts and refers to the idea that you should be able to present your "message" in the time it would take to ride in an elevator. As you are working on your communication strategies, be sure to include the development of an elevator speech in case you need to meet with potential funders, school boards, or others who simply want to understand the key points of your project.

Caregiver training and professional development. As part of your plan implementation, your team begins to consider the different types of training and professional development that will be implemented. You have two broad efforts in this category: educating caregivers and providing professional development to teachers. Included in this training are ideas about how to decrease children's fears, strategies for reassuring children, and ways to have low-cost fun as a family. Your team decides to provide these trainings through the parent volunteers who will host these trainings in community venues. The school psychologist, school counselor, and a therapist from the local mental health agency work together to develop the content of these workshops and to train the parent volunteers. Additionally, they work together to develop brief newsletter articles and flyers for families who are unable to attend.

In the school, the school psychologist, school counselor, principal, and teacher representatives work together to plan the professional development around the school-wide PBIS program at Ansel Adams. As noted, the program was originally developed and implemented but had fallen by the wayside over the years. As the team examines the existing program, they decide that it needs some updating. They plan to hold a series of whole school meetings so that all teachers and staff can participate in updating this program. Through this process, they plan to increase teacher knowledge of PBIS and increase investment in the program. The final planning meetings will include developing a strategy for implementation and forming a school-based PBIS team that will be responsible for helping integrate aspects of the program throughout the school.

KEY STEPS IN PLAN IMPLEMENTATION

- Develop an intervention plan with your group based on your knowledge, research, and available resources.
  - Decide on the level(s) of intervention that you will provide.
  - Be sure your plans are well defined in terms of goals, outcomes, timelines, and implementation. This step helps to ensure fidelity.

- Determine the order in which you will implement your plan.
- Begin an outline of your logic model based on your intervention plan that includes inputs (i.e., resources) and activities (i.e., prevention programming).
- Communicate your plan with school personnel, families, and community members.
  - Try to reach as many individuals as possible.
  - If you are seeking funding from community agencies, be sure you can communicate your message quickly and in a compelling manner.
- Provide professional development and caregiver training.

STAGE 5: MONITORING AND EVALUATING OUTCOMES

After your working groups have identified the goals for each of the various programs, you define the *outputs* for your logic model. That is, your team identifies the types of outcomes that you expect to see as the result of your efforts. In addition to defining those specific outcomes, you also want to determine the data sources that will be used to decide whether your plan was effective. You do not want to spend a great deal of time, effort, and resources on programs that are not effective. Together, the team develops a comprehensive, yet practical, evaluation and monitoring plan. Figure 9.3 outlines the complete logic model with the expected outcomes and the methods for evaluating each aspect of the overall plan.

The plan involves periodic ongoing measures of the risk and protective factors reported previously, along with monitoring of levels of behavioral concerns noted at Ansel Adams Elementary School. Additionally, formative evaluations of intervention implementation and integrity are conducted to ensure that the programs are being implemented with fidelity. The team also identifies the types of outcomes that they expect to see in the short term (e.g., increased implementation of consistent discipline) and the medium term (e.g., improved levels of behavior). Some of the long-term indicators are not written into this plan but might include improved teacher satisfaction and ongoing maintenance of positive outcomes such as continuing improvement in grades, behavior, and parent involvement.

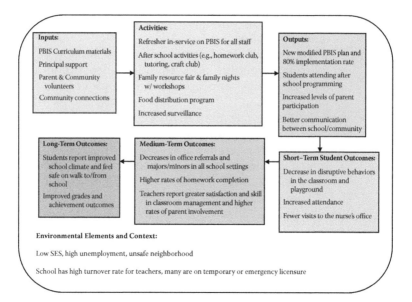

Figure 9.3 Ansel Adams program evaluation logic model.

- Identify outcomes for each aspect of your program.
  - Be sure to include evaluation of process components such as the degree to which the plan was implemented as intended and the success of your communication plan in reaching the intended audience.
- Identify appropriate outcome measures or indicators to determine whether your program is having the intended effect.
- Monitor progress at different points.
- Consider the short-term, medium-term, and long-term outcomes that you would expect to see after successful plan implementation.

CONCLUSION

We purposely selected a more complicated case to outline the steps in the Public Health Problem-Solving Model to demonstrate the ways that this process can be used to address very

difficult problems. If the concerns in a given school represented a single focus or concern, the process would be more
straightforward. As with all processes, these steps (CD 9.2)
serve as guidelines to help guide your team. You may find that
you make adaptations along the way to best meet the needs of
your system. As you read through this case study, maybe you
were thinking about the aspects of this work that were similar
to what you already are doing in your system. Likewise, you
may be thinking how different some of these tasks are from
your current role as a school psychologist. As noted throughout this text, the implementation of this model includes find-
ing a balance between aspects of your current role, but also
incorporating a preventive, broad-based focus for addressing
complex problems such as meeting the mental health needs
of children.

Ten

Changing Role of
School Psychologists

In contrast to clinical models, expertise in pathology and assessment are not the crucial skills for providing comprehensive children's mental health services. Because the Public Health Problem-Solving Model will lead to many programs that are delivered at the classroom and systemic levels, the level of expertise can be broad and applied to any individual who knows the curriculum and who is skilled in program delivery components (e.g., classroom management). What this means is that teachers, school counselors, social workers, school psychologists, and, in some cases, paraprofessionals may all be adequately prepared to deliver many, if not all, of the program components.

With the public health model, we are giving psychology away to those who can have the broadest impact on the greatest number of individuals. This thinking represents a shift; in some ways, it is exciting and in other ways, frightening. What will be our unique role in this new model? Will we make ourselves obsolete? Again, our message is that the Public Health Problem-Solving Model will not replace what we are doing: It will be a supplemental component to our efforts in the schools. It represents a means for maximizing our services by shifting our focus from intervention to prevention and health promotion.

APPLYING SCHOOL PSYCHOLOGY SKILLS
TO COMPREHENSIVE CHILDREN'S
MENTAL HEALTH SERVICES

Although adopting the Public Health Problem-Solving Model to the practice of psychology in the schools is a paradigm shift, there are many aspects of traditional school psychology that can be easily revised to support a public health practice of school psychology. These skill sets include the following:

- Utilizing the problem-solving model to provide comprehensive children's mental health services
- Utilizing data-driven decision-making so that the appropriate comprehensive children's mental health issues are addressed
- Utilizing appropriate evidence-based interventions so that appropriate comprehensive children's mental health services are provided, and collecting and interpreting local data so that outcomes from comprehensive children's mental health services can be evaluated
- Utilizing consultation and collaboration to support the implementation of comprehensive children's mental health services

Utilizing the Public Health Problem-Solving Model to provide comprehensive children's mental health services. School psychologists understand the utility of the problem-solving model and how to guide others through this model. The Response to Intervention movement and much individual consultation is based on the problem-solving model. As we adopt a comprehensive public health model, it is helpful to remind ourselves and others that this is what we have been doing at the individual level, now taken to a community level.

Utilizing data-driven decision-making so that the appropriate comprehensive children's mental health issues are addressed. School psychologists are experts at utilizing data to drive interventions. We conduct behavioral observations, interview others, evaluate permanent products, and review records to develop a functional behavioral analysis (FBA). Based on this FBA, we explain to others how we can restructure the environment to increase the likelihood that a student is engaging in appropriate behavior. We utilize standardized and individualized assessments to determine a student's range of proximal development. From this information, we work with others to refine curriculum and instructional methods to scaffold a student's development.

These techniques and skills, which have been utilized with individual students, are transferable to a population-based public health practice of school psychology. For most identified issues, there will be national data and norms. Very likely, there will not be local data and norms. As outlined in previous chapters, local data must be collected to establish incidence and prevalence rates for populations and subpopulations. Then we must create an FBA for the populations of interest and agree how to alter the environment so that positive trajectories are supported and negative trajectories are altered. Again, it will be important that school psychologists recognize and publicize how their skills are applicable to population-based problem-solving.

Utilizing appropriate evidence-based interventions so that appropriate comprehensive children's mental health services are provided, and collecting and interpreting local data so that outcomes from comprehensive children's mental health services can be evaluated. Data-driven decision-making is a recursive loop. We utilize data to understand the baseline and select an evidence-based intervention. However, we then continue to collect data to assess the fidelity of implementation as well as student outcomes, intended and unintended. It is critical that we do not repeat the errors of DARE, where anti-drug programming was shown at best to have no lasting effect (Lyman et al., 1999). More prevalent in education is the adoption of glossy products with no outcome data or solutions-of-the-month, trendy solutions that oversimplify challenges.

As research-based practitioners, we understand the need to critically assess possible interventions. Our training has shown us that complex, multi-determined behaviors will not be quickly eradicated with superficial poultices. Our position in the schools also gives us more autonomy to question politically driven or ill-thought-out interventions. Similarly, we know that carefully selected well-thought-out interventions, delivered with fidelity and matched to needs, can greatly increase the capacity of school systems and their partners to address the mental health needs of all students (Merrell & Buchanan, 2006).

Utilizing consultation and collaboration to support the implementation of comprehensive children's mental health services. A strong theme throughout this book has been that population-based change will require multiple players working in concert. School psychologists are trained to provide consultation. Consultation is the art and science of convincing other people to change for the good of someone else or something else. Instructional consultation has been defined as having three central elements: (1) the problem-solving stages, (2) the communication and relationship with the consultee, and (3) the use of evidence-based assessments and interventions

(Rosenfield, 2008). Utilizing the problem-solving stages, attending to our relationships and communication with all stakeholders, and utilizing evidence-based assessments and interventions to guide our work is exactly what is prescribed in a public health model of mental health provision. Again, recognizing the transferability of our existing skills and making administrators or community members aware of our abilities to facilitate change are critical to our success.

PROFESSIONAL AND LEGAL IMPERATIVES TO UTILIZE A COMPREHENSIVE MENTAL HEALTH MODEL IN OUR WORK

In Table 10.1, we have listed typical activities of school psychology training and practice that might be associated with each dimension of traditional practice. We then provide examples of training and practice that also correspond to competency domains of school psychology but that broaden the focus of school psychology to include practice with systems and populations. The form in CD 10.1 can be used for planning change in your own practice. As noted in Chapter 1, the movement toward more systemic, preventive models is consistent with the new model of comprehensive services promoted by NASP. It seems clear that school psychologists' skill set generalizes easily from individual practice to public practice, and that these two service delivery modes actually comprise complementary frameworks for ensuring comprehensive services to children and their families.

As you consider your first steps in adopting this practice, we also provide some cautions. Practitioners who attempt to implement too many new programs and initiate additional projects may quickly find themselves overwhelmed. Unfortunately, they may become burned out and cynical to the possibility of change. We address some of the risks of taking on too much without considering your priorities and a realistic appraisal of your ability to implement aspects of this model in your current setting.

AVOIDING BURNOUT

Even if the Public Health Problem-Solving Model is within the existing skill set of most school psychologists, it still requires additional work and time. As stated before, we argue

Table 10.1 Comparison of Traditional and Expanded Domains of NASP-Identified School Psychology Training and Practice

NASP Domain	Traditional Practice (Addressing Individuals With Problems)	Expanded Public Health Practice (Addressing Prevention, Populations, and Systems)	Comments
Data-Based Decision-Making and Accountability School psychologists have knowledge of varied models and methods of assessment and data collection methods for identifying strengths and needs, developing effective services and programs, and measuring progress and outcomes.	**Existing Areas** Assessment of: • Cognitive abilities • Social–emotional functioning • Behavior • Achievement • Classroom environments	**Existing Areas** • Assisting with efforts to gather achievement data on all students (e.g., curriculum-based assessment, progress monitoring). **Potential Areas** • Assessment of the extent, incidence, and/or prevalence of school and community issues (e.g., dropping out, violence, differential achievement in minorities, etc.) • Assessment of risk and protective factors in prevention/promotion programs • Assessment of program implementation and outcomes for various subpopulations	This domain underlies school psychology practice and training. Historically, it has been a clinical area as almost all of our focus has been on individual assessment of children with problems. Because administrators and decision-makers typically need data to address school and community problems, opportunities for expansion are likely to appear in numerous school systems.

Continued

Table 10.1 (continued) Comparison of Traditional and Expanded Domains of NASP-Identified School Psychology Training and Practice

NASP Domain	Traditional Practice (Addressing Individuals With Problems)	Expanded Public Health Practice (Addressing Prevention, Populations, and Systems)	Comments
Consultation and Collaboration School psychologists have knowledge of varied models and strategies of consultation, collaboration, and communication applicable to individuals, families, groups, and systems and methods to promote effective implementation of services.	**Existing Areas** Generally the focus has been on one student at a time through: • Client-centered case consultation • Consultee-centered case consultation • Collaboration and didactic professional development	**Existing Areas** • Organizational and systems consultation **Potential Areas** • Expanded focus on systems consultation • Interagency collaboration • Comprehensive service delivery • "Trainer of trainer" models, where school psychologists coach other professionals, paraprofessionals, and volunteers in group intervention provision	A second traditional strength of school psychology, again primarily focused on individual children with problems. Although much has been written about comprehensive services, training for and practice of such services remain less common.

Interventions and Instructional Support to Develop Academic Skills

School psychologists have knowledge of biological, cultural, and social influences on academic skills; human learning, cognitive, and developmental processes; and evidence-based curricula and instructional strategies.

Existing Areas

- Using educational data to help develop or select interventions on school problem-solving teams.
- Supporting students' development of access skills (e.g., study skills, attention, memory)

Existing Areas

- Assisting with the implementation of classroom management and PBIS[a] models to help students spend more time academically engaged.

Potential Areas

- Development of school and district mechanisms to track effectiveness of whole-student programming on academic outcomes
- Longitudinal analysis of student outcomes and early risk indicators

A third traditional area of emphasis in school psychology, although historically targeted at individual children once problems have developed. In contrast to the two previously mentioned areas, relatively less emphasis has occurred in school psychology on educational interventions (as opposed to assessment).

Continued

Table 10.1 (continued)   Comparison of Traditional and Expanded Domains of NASP-Identified School Psychology Training and Practice

NASP Domain	Traditional Practice (Addressing Individuals With Problems)	Expanded Public Health Practice (Addressing Prevention, Populations, and Systems)	Comments
Interventions and Mental Health Services to Develop Social and Life Skills School psychologists have knowledge of biological, cultural, developmental, and social influences on behavior and mental health, behavioral, and emotional impacts on learning and life skills, and evidence-based strategies to promote social–emotional functioning and mental health.	**Existing Areas** Focus has tended to be on one student at a time: • Behavioral interventions • Individual counseling • Group counseling • Social skills training • Case consultation	**Existing Areas** • Delivery of school- or class-wide social skills curricula • Small group counseling for students with identified targeted needs or increased risk factors **Potential Areas** • Increased reliance on prevention science to develop whole school programming • Development of collaborative networks with community agencies • Increased public education regarding the mental health needs of students • Professional development through in-service programs to school staff • Program monitoring and evaluation • Ongoing advocacy	This area has significant applications in public practice. Historically, it has been applied to direct and indirect psychological interventions for individual children.

School-Wide Practices to Promote Learning

School psychologists have knowledge of school and systems structure, organization, and theory; general and special education; technology resources; and evidence-based school practices that promote learning and mental health.

Existing Areas

- Understanding of schools as systems
- Participation in school improvement or building leadership teams

Existing Areas

- Understanding of students as existing in many interrelated ecologies (family, school, community, etc.)
- Wraparound services for students with intensive needs

Potential Areas

- Building liaisons between family, school, and community groups to coordinate service provision efforts at all levels of the prevention continuum
- Professional development with multiple stakeholders and service providers
- Policy development and analysis
- Advocacy with decision-makers and stakeholders
- Consultation and transfer of psychological knowledge and expertise
- Empowerment and facilitation of communication

Within school psychology, implementation of this domain largely has emphasized the first part of the description: knowledge and understanding of schools as systems. The second part, policy development and advocacy for system improvement, requires a public health model.

Continued

Table 10.1 (continued)   Comparison of Traditional and Expanded Domains of NASP-Identified School Psychology Training and Practice

NASP Domain	Traditional Practice (Addressing Individuals With Problems)	Expanded Public Health Practice (Addressing Prevention, Populations, and Systems)	Comments
Preventive and Responsive Services School psychologists have knowledge of principles and research related to resilience and risk factors in learning and mental health, services in schools and communities to support multi-tiered prevention, and evidence-based strategies for effective crisis response.	**Existing Areas** • Application of risk and resiliency factors to student demographics • Participation in prevention efforts (e.g., implementation of school-wide programs such as PBIS and RtI[b]) • Crisis planning and response	**Existing Areas** • Small-group, school-based secondary prevention activities • School-wide secondary prevention programs (e.g., violence prevention) • Referral of students and families to community resources **Potential Areas** • Prevention science (identification, assessment, and management of risk and protective factors associated with educational, health, and mental health outcomes) • Educating the public about prevention • Advocacy and policy development • Integrated and comprehensive prevention and intervention • Empowerment of students and families • Monitoring and program evaluation	This is a public practice domain, although it is difficult to understand how these three distinct areas are grouped conceptually into a single domain. Existing activities in this domain seem to emphasize school-based secondary prevention projects.

Family-School Collaboration Services	Existing Areas	Existing Areas	
School psychologists have knowledge of principles and research related to family systems, strengths, needs, and culture; evidence-based strategies to support family influences on children's learning and mental health; and strategies to develop collaboration between families and schools.	• Parent/family involvement in assessments • Parent/family interventions	• In-service training • Conjoint consultation **Potential Areas** • Services integration through integration and collaboration with community service providers • Empowerment of families through home-school linkages that promote two-way communication • Educating the public about school- and student-related issues • Monitoring of attitudes and participation among families and community agencies • Policy development and advocacy • Program evaluation	This domain has been difficult for schools and communities (much less school psychologists) to implement, in part because policies, attitudes, trust, and involvement likely must precede practice. Use of a public health model with an emphasis on empowerment may help promote true collaboration and partnership.

Continued

Table 10.1 (continued) Comparison of Traditional and Expanded Domains of NASP-Identified School Psychology Training and Practice

NASP Domain	Traditional Practice (Addressing Individuals With Problems)	Expanded Public Health Practice (Addressing Prevention, Populations, and Systems)	Comments
Diversity in Development and Learning School psychologists have knowledge of individual differences, abilities, disabilities, and other diverse characteristics; principles and research related to diversity factors for children, families, and schools, including factors related to culture, context, and individual and role differences; and evidence-based strategies to enhance services and address potential influences related to diversity.	**Existing Areas** • Advocacy for individual students • Cultural sensitivity in clinical practice	**Existing Areas** • Professional development for faculty on cultural competency **Potential Areas** • Educating public about diversity issues in development and learning • Policy development and advocacy • Promotion of social justice and equity of educational opportunities • Analyzing program implementation and evaluation data to ensure equal access and outcomes	This domain is framed to address the needs and characteristics of individual students. Nonetheless, diversity represents a significant challenge for schools and communities as systems. Helping these systems address issues of diversity likely will require a public model.

Research and Program Evaluation

School psychologists have knowledge of research design, statistics, measurement, varied data collection and analysis techniques, and program evaluation sufficient for understanding research and interpreting data in applied settings.

Existing Areas
- Single-subject research
- Intervention accountability
- Evaluation of behavior plans or small projects

Existing Areas
- Group research design

Potential Areas
- Program evaluation
- Monitoring student mental health through epidemiology
- Prevention science
- Development of logic models
- Integrating parents, students, and others into program evaluation efforts

As in the case of the first domain, this is an overarching domain. However, a clear conceptual and practical distinction between clinical research and public health activities (e.g., prevention and program evaluation) would highlight applications related to public practice.

Legal, Ethical, and Professional Practice

School psychologists have knowledge of the history and foundations of school psychology; multiple service models and methods; ethical, legal, and professional standards; and other factors related to professional identity and effective practice as school psychologists.

Existing Areas
- Involvement in professional organizations
- Legal and ethical practice
- Professional development

Existing Areas
- Rights of children protected through NCLB[c], IDEA[d], and other legislation

Potential Areas
- Policy development and advocacy
- Assist problem-solving teams in utilization of supports and student outcomes
- Monitoring program outputs and outcomes

This is an overarching domain, but seems primarily to focus on within-profession identity and function rather than on public practice.

a PBIS: Positive Behavioral Interventions and Supports.
b RtI: Response to Interventions.
c NCLB: No Child Left Behind.
d IDEA: Individuals with Disabilities Education Act.

that utilization of the Public Health Problem-Solving Model should expand rather than replace traditional school psychology practice. So, how do you find the time to practice in this way? There are four components that we think are critical:

- Examining your workload
- Sharing the work with others
- Starting small
- Taking care of yourself

Examining your workload. As George Sugai said when introducing Positive Behavioral Interventions and Supports (PBIS) to a group of Colorado educators in 1990s, "What are you not going to do?" There was a shocked silence in the audience: The world would end if we stopped doing any of our critical work. He went on to explain that everyone in the room was contributing more to their work than was probably optimal for their health and private life; if they were going to add the implementation of PBIS to their schools and districts, they were going to have to stop doing something that they currently were doing.

Ideally, you would receive a release from some of your current duties to implement comprehensive mental health services, but that may not happen for all of us. If not (or not initially), you will have to decide which of your current duties can be done by someone else or not done for a while.

One means to increase efficiency is to integrate the work of providing comprehensive children's mental health services into existing programs or committees. For instance, some schools' Response to Intervention (RtI) teams are only (or predominantly) focused on individual students. However, the RtI model is directly aligned with the public health approach and addresses all levels of need. Expanding this committee to proactively encompass universal, targeted, and intensive interventions would require additional work and collaboration but could be more effective and less time-intensive than creating an additional committee. Similarly a district-level team that supports schools in Tier 3 behavioral interventions could be expanded to consider how all children in the district might be better supported in their social and behavioral development. Ultimately the enhanced primary and secondary services will decrease the tertiary needs and referrals. However, initially, workload will increase, and so it is important to consider how you will juggle this.

Sharing the work with others. Successfully addressing all children's mental health needs will take the whole village. Change is most effective when you start with people who want to work toward a common goal; gradually, the naysayers either join with the movement or move away. Peer support will not only make the work manageable for you, it also has the potential to change the norms of the system so that preventative innovations receive greater support (Rogers, 2002). So, start with a couple of individuals who share your commitment: people with whom you can share the work, people who hold each other accountable and support each other when the going gets tough. As Margaret Mead (n.d.) is so often quoted as saying, "Never doubt that a small group of thoughtful, committed citizens can change the world. Indeed, it's the only thing that ever has."

Starting small. Often when we start collecting data on a social or mental health issue, we can feel overwhelmed by the enormity of the needs. The reason that many individuals do not acknowledge pervasive and serious problems may be a sense of inadequacy in their abilities to address them. Denial is a powerful coping mechanism but not an effective long-term strategy for change. At the same time, it is important to realize that you were not the creator of the identified problem, you will not be able to change it alone, and change takes more time than usually expected. A small success is much more useful to everyone than a large failure. A small success can create momentum and larger, longer commitments. So instead of tackling child poverty initially, it may make more sense to address decreasing the number of F's at the ninth-grade level at one high school. This may lead to the provision of more academic and extracurricular after school activities. This may lead to higher high school graduation rates and post-secondary training success. Ultimately, these students are able to be better providers for their future families. Voilà, decreased child poverty rates! Even though you are starting small, it is critical to have a conceptual model of causation, change, and implementation that considers your unique context; otherwise, any change that occurs will either not be noticed or not be attributable to your efforts (Shapiro, 2006).

Taking care of yourself. We recognize and respect that implementing the Public Health Problem-Solving Model in schools and communities is difficult work. You are a critical element in this formula and if you do not keep yourself invigorated, you and all those whom you could have positively affected will suffer. A lot of training and practice is required to develop as a school psychologist; this is not to be taken lightly. The Public Health Problem-Solving Model can lead to amazing successes, vibrant coalitions, and significant impacts for many people you may never meet. And that can be just the problem for our continued commitment: people you may never meet. Most of us entered school psychology because we wanted to work directly with students and to see that our time spent with them led to improved outcomes in their lives. In this model, you get to work primarily with adults and the results can be nebulous, or at least distant. On top of that, change can be slow and nonlinear. For every advance, there may be multiple setbacks. Prevention is notoriously difficult to measure (Rogers, 2002), and, even if you can confidently calculate a change in teen pregnancy rates, there is no face to attach to the increased percentage of students who didn't become parents.

For all these reasons, it is imperative that you consciously and consistently attend to taking care of yourself. The first step is to find a supportive community. Some of these people may be partners in the work. It is also helpful to have supportive peers outside of your immediate work, who value what you are attempting: local or remote colleagues, who can understand your struggles and remind you of your successes when you are having trouble remembering them.

This is the second important practice: Celebrate successes along the way. Regular public celebrations should be scheduled to recognize what has been accomplished, to honor those who have done the work, and to promote the next steps. This reflection and public acknowledgment is important for empowering the persons involved in the work (Cattaneo & Chapman, 2010), as well as to continue to receive external support (Sugai & Horner, 2006).

Finally, it is a long road. You will only stay on the path if you have a clear vision for what you are trying to accomplish and you periodically revisit and refine that vision. A personal belief system in which you value all children and believe that positive outcomes are possible for all students is required; strengths-based (see, e.g., Maton et al., 2004) and positive psychology (see, e.g., Gilman, Huebner, & Furlong, 2009) research can help bolster that belief system. Although this work may not lead to many hugs from kids in the hall, we know it can keep more kids in school, and that is work worth doing!

CONCLUSION

Practicing from a public health paradigm is difficult work: It forces you to face the inequities and injustices in the world. It is also a paradigm that gives you the tools to promote social justice and opportunities for all students. Although you have the skills required to practice in this manner, you may have to shift how you apply these skills as you promote a preventative, holistic approach to psychology in the schools. This form of practice is in keeping with professional standards and legal mandates. However, as you begin to practice the Public Health Problem-Solving Model that provides comprehensive mental health services for all students, you will face obstacles. For yourself and the clients you serve, it is imperative that you promote your own mental health and avoid burnout.

Eleven

Sustaining Change
in the Public Health
Problem-Solving Model

L ong-term prevention and intervention programs rely
on systems that are able to support and sustain these
efforts. Unfortunately, those who lead research projects
and grant funded initiatives sometimes do not address the
underlying foundations of systems change. By combining your
knowledge of problem-solving and a public health model, you
can create sustainable processes that help to ensure that
your efforts do not end with the current school year.

MAINTAINING SYSTEMS CHANGE

We have come a long way in our understanding of how to
implement systems change. Still, findings from early work
in this area are applicable today. For example, Hightower,
Johnson, and Haffey (1995) conceptualized the process of program adoption in the schools as requiring three stages: planning and preparation, implementation, and maintenance. Our
model of change—the Public Health Problem-Solving Model—
has a similar progression of stages, but we have defined each
stage in more depth (Chapters 4 through 8) so that it can be
used to guide your efforts at addressing a single issue of concern, or to create broader change as presented in our case
study (Chapter 9). We now address the issue of maintenance.
How do you facilitate the conditions that will help keep your
efforts moving forward?

The desired end result for your team's efforts is sustained
systems change. However, as noted early on, true change is
very difficult. In this chapter, we address some of the broader
foundational issues that must also be in place to help you

persist in your efforts over time. Whether it occurs through ongoing monitoring, advocacy, research dissemination, or influencing policy and legislation, the results of our efforts should be sustained and meaningful.

Ongoing Monitoring

If we have found success in our programming efforts, it is tempting to assume that we have solved the problem and no longer need to attend to that specific issue. You have built monitoring into your logic model that will allow you to address your short- and medium-term outcomes, but sometimes it can be difficult to measure the longer term outcomes. These types of goals can sometimes be more difficult to monitor (e.g., increased parent satisfaction with the school, more positive school environment). Therefore, when our short-term goals are met, we sometimes believe that our long-term outcomes will unfold as well.

As you finalize your logic model and program evaluation plan, your team will want to ensure that you have built in long-term monitoring, even though your plan has been adopted, is fully implemented, and appears to be working. Unfortunately, changes in leadership, new priorities, and resource reallocations are all potential threats that could derail your efforts. Therefore, ongoing monitoring is needed to determine whether your program is continuing to be implemented in the manner in which it was planned.

Within a school setting, there is a certain amount of turnover each year with new teachers, administrators, and students entering the system. You may find that after a year or two, many of your original supporters have moved on, and it is only through ongoing professional development and advocacy that you can maintain the momentum and support for your program. By monitoring awareness of and attitudes toward the issues, you can be alert to when additional efforts are needed by the coalition to recruit new members, disseminate information, or provide continuing professional development opportunities.

Advocacy

Advocacy will be a part of your role at each step as you are implementing the Public Health Problem-Solving Model. School psychologists are expected to advocate for students and families as outlined in the most recent version of the NASP Professional Ethics, adopted in January 2011. Unfortunately, there is not a great deal in the school psychology literature about advocacy and "how to" advocate. We view advocacy as part of your sustained efforts to make ongoing positive changes in your school system.

> The child deserves an advocate to represent him and his needs to the society in which he lives, an advocate who will insist that programs and services based on sound child development knowledge will be available to every child as a public utility—the promotion of national, state, and community responsibility and initiative in developing comprehensive and systematic programs of prevention and treatment, in increasing the accountability of those who [ad]minister relevant programs, and in coordinating and organizing resources for supportive, effective, and coordinated programs for our children and youth. (Joint Commission on Mental Health of Children, 1970, p. 9).

This statement represents both a beginning and an end point of your efforts. Your first step as an advocate is simply to become involved. As you look around your school or community, you can see any number of opportunities for positive change. However, when you make the psychological commitment to dedicate time and effort to a particular issue, you have made your first step as an advocate. Later steps may include your work to create positive, prevention programming for youth, as the final product, whether it is through the implementation of a new program, more effective district policies, or greater public awareness and a working coalition. Each of these outcomes reflects *advocacy*, or acting on behalf of, youth and their families. Moreover, your efforts are carried out in a systematic and purposeful manner with the goal of changing a situation (Gibelman & Kraft, 1996).

Advocacy, by its nature, involves risk. When we strongly speak up for a position, a program, or a child, we place ourselves at risk. How can that be, you might ask? Isn't advocacy a good thing and part of my role? Of course it is, but it comes with potential dangers. For one, when we advocate for one position, we might distance ourselves from someone who holds a different perspective. If we advocate too vigorously, the chance for losing support is increased (Berkowitz & Wolff, 2000). Therefore, it is always important to proceed with caution and to understand the issues before you go forward.

Knitzer (1976), a long-standing advocate for children's mental health, outlined the following fundamental assumptions of advocacy:

1. People have, or ought to have, certain basic rights.
2. These rights are enforceable by statutory, administrative, or judicial procedures.
3. Advocacy is focused on institutional failures that produce or aggravate individual problems.
4. Advocacy is inherently political.
5. Advocacy is most effective when it is focused on specific issues.
6. Advocacy is different from provision of direct services.

In reflecting back on her long career, Knitzer (2005) described her three main strategies as to always look at issues through "multiple lenses," to join with others, and to link her efforts with public policy, either directly or by influencing those who were in a position to effect policy. As you are working with your team and planning for change, you are likely engaging in these first two strategies. However, as a group, consider whether there are policies that might need to be changed with your prevention planning (discussed in more depth later in this chapter).

Persuasion and Negotiation

From the beginning, your team will be engaging in advocacy. As noted, your decision to attend to an issue is the first step. However, the next greatest challenge will be to encourage others to act. Hoefer (2006) describes two of the greatest advocacy skills as persuasion and negotiation. From the beginning, persuasion occurs when you convince others that taking action and, ultimately, implementing your coalition's plan of action is in their best interest. To accomplish this task, you will need to lay the groundwork, which entails preparing members, collecting facts, and sharing this information with others (Berkowitz & Wolff, 2000).

The second skill, negotiation, reflects a basic form of communication that we use all of the time. When we state a position or a request, it is rare that we get exactly what we ask for, so we learn to propose alternatives or set priorities until all parties involved in the conversation are satisfied with the outcome. Negotiation might occur around something as simple as when to set a meeting. At other times, it may reflect a much more complex exchange. When negotiating, you will want to have your absolute limits in mind, as well as your priorities, so that you can more readily maintain focus on those issues that must be addressed and allow those that are secondary to your overall goal to be tabled, if needed.

Research dissemination. As noted, the act of persuasion will occur throughout your efforts, from the moment you convince your principal to support the development of a planning team to the point where you share the results of your work with others. We have covered many of the aspects of persuasion in earlier chapters. For example, when you invite members to be involved in a problem-solving process, when you share data related to the issue of concern, and when you educate others about the particular issue, you are using forms of persuasion. In this chapter, we focus on the form of persuasion that occurs when you want to share your work with others.

Often the idea of "sharing your findings with others" is not incorporated into practitioner-oriented resources. Conversely, we believe that disseminating your findings with others serves an important educational function by helping others to solve difficult problems of practice. In some ways, your work might persuade others to adopt a new practice or try a more effective approach in their own settings. Your findings are also important to administrators, potential funding sources, and community supporters who will be making important policy, resource allocation, or involvement decisions related to your work. Each of these components has important implications for sustainability.

There are three main audiences with whom you will want to share your findings: scholars, those who work in professional settings, and participants in your project (Bellmore & Graham, 2009). Although we recognize the importance of sharing your findings in a traditional format through publication and presentation at conferences, we also recognize that it is not always possible because of time and cost constraints. Instead, we focus on professionals and participants as the two key audiences.

The first group, those who work in professional settings, represent individuals who have the potential to implement these changes in their own settings and to support resulting policy development (i.e., practitioners, principals, superintendents, policy-makers). Your team will want to consider some of the most efficient methods for disseminating information to reach key members of this audience. For example, if you want to share your work with other school psychology practitioners, a logical outlet is a state professional conference. The same format may be used to disseminate your work with other professionals as well. You may partner with your school administration, teachers, or other service providers (e.g., school counselor, agency therapist) to present to their respective state organizations. Also consider writing brief articles for professional newsletters across different disciplines.

Reaching policy-makers at the community level can sometimes be more difficult. However, consider inviting local representatives to your information sharing sessions, write articles or opinion editorial pieces for the local paper, and send your key findings to school board members, city council representatives, and educational representatives at the state level. Through these efforts, you will be more likely to "catch" the attention of individuals who may be in a position to help support your program efforts.

Those who have participated in your program are also a key audience because their lives have been directly impacted by your prevention efforts. During planned family nights at school (e.g., parent–teacher conferences, back-to-school night), create a display and a brief presentation that shares your findings with family members. Be sure to consider methods for integrating family voice and decision-making into your dissemination efforts as well. Family volunteers can help with the presentations and can also help decide on other audiences with whom they would like to share the results.

Influencing policy and legislation. As with persuasion, negotiation will also have been an integral part of your practice since the initial formation of your work group. In fact, we would suggest that school psychologists are especially skilled at the art of negotiation because of the frequent mediating role that they play in their schools. Your work in the Public Health Problem-Solving Model will involve negotiating with your principal, your coalition members, and many others.

At the broadest levels, one way to increase sustainability is to advocate for policy and legislative changes that support your programming. At this point, you may not view your efforts as directed toward changing public policy, but it is possible that through your efforts you may come to realize that a specific school policy acts as a barrier to family involvement or creates unequal access to programming. In those instances, part of your team's longer term strategy may involve working to modify a specific school or district policy. In this way, you are influencing local educational policies and practices.

The first step in influencing policy is establishing communication with policy-makers. If you live in a small community, it might be possible to simply invite these individuals to your planning or information sharing sessions. In larger communities, it is not as easy. Groark and McCall (2005) suggest writing a briefing paper that provides a detailed but concise (no more than one page) outline of an identified problem and solution. In this case, the concern identified at your school, your prevention plan, and the outcomes of your efforts would constitute the body of this briefing paper. Additionally, look for opportunities in the community such as forums, planning groups, or other venues where policy-makers may be present to share the work of your team.

Once you have established this communication, be sure that you keep your request clear and succinct. What policy do you want to see implemented and why? How would you like to see a policy changed and why? As noted in the chapter on ecological plan implementation (Chapter 7), you want to stick to the evidence. With your logic model and your outcome data, it will be easy for your team to establish the support for a specific position. Your team may want to focus on one policy change at a time. It can be overwhelming to be approached with multiple requests for adding new policies, changing existing ones, and deleting others. As you move forward, keep in mind that your ultimate goal is to improve the mental health and well-being of children.

Maintaining and sustaining the vitality of your coalition over time may be one of the more difficult aspects of this work. Coalitions can get sidetracked, bogged down on an issue, or simply run out of steam. Some of the ways that you can avoid these pitfalls is to have a sufficient number of members who can share the work and are invested in an identified issue. Once your coalition appears to have sufficiently addressed the issue at hand, you may find that your group wants to change its focus, cut back, come to an end, or simply remain the same. Your group will want to consider what is needed to maintain the programming that was set into motion, but it does not always mean that the coalition will be the responsible party. Ideally, the involved systems (e.g., school, community agencies) will have taken over their own components of the programming. One of the components that will help to sustain a coalition, especially when members are tired or frustrated, is the belief in the value of what you are doing. (Use CD 11.1 to reflect on your efforts.) In the next paragraphs, we return to the idea of why it is important to change our current ways of addressing the mental health needs of students.

Social Justice Perspective

We began this text with the idea (cited by Beauchamp, 1976) that public health was a form of social justice. We would add to this idea by noting that prevention also provides a framework for promoting social justice (Kenny, Horne, Orpinas, & Reese, 2009). The term *social justice* has a long history and is defined in many different ways. In their survey of school psychologists who were experts in the area of cultural diversity, Shriberg et al. (2008) attempted to identify the meaning of social justice from a school psychology perspective. They found that participants most often endorsed the definition of social justice that included "ensuring the protection of rights and responsibilities for all" (p. 461). Within this global definition is the idea of equal access to appropriate services.

School psychologists have a long history of advocating for the rights of students through support of equal access policies in school, upholding ideals of nondiscriminatory practices, and acting as change agents within the school setting (Sheridan & Gutkin, 2000; Shriberg et al., 2008). We view the implementation of a Public Health Problem-Solving Model as an effective framework for addressing complex problems in school settings, many of which may be related to issues of inequality. This model is consistent with the ideal that school psychologists engage in advocacy for students that supports their rights and opportunities (Shriberg et al., 2008). We also expand on this position by suggesting that through the development of a representative, empowered coalition, we can overcome economic and institutional barriers rather than simply acknowledge their presence.

CONCLUSION

We can no longer afford to have separate programs within schools and communities that are structurally and philosophically independent. Instead, we should direct our efforts toward developing seamless supports that identify and support the academic, social, and emotional needs of children. Using our skills as school psychologists, we can build coalitions that allow us to impact broader problems of practice. The Public Health Problem-Solving Model represents a promising avenue for guiding our efforts toward positive systemic change.

References

Abramson, L.Y., Alloy, L. B., Hankin, B. L., Haeffel, G. J., MacCoon, D. G., & Gibb, B. E. (2002). Cognitive vulnerability-stress models of depression in a self-regulatory and psychobiological context. In I. H. Gotlib & C. I. Hammen (Eds.), *Handbook of depression* (pp. 268–294). New York: Guilford Press.

Adelman, H. S., & Taylor, L. (2000). Looking at school health and school reform policy through the lens of addressing barriers to learning. Children's services. *Social Policy, Research, and Practice, 3*(2), 117–132.

Adelman, H. S., & Taylor, L. (2003). On sustainability of project innovations as systemic change. *Journal of Educational and Psychological Consultation, 14*, 1–26.

Adelman, H. S., & Taylor, L. (2009). Ending the marginalization of mental health in schools: A comprehensive approach. In R. W. Christner & R. B. Mennuti (Eds.), *School-based mental health: A practitioner's guide to comparative practices* (pp. 25–54). New York: Routledge.

Adelman, H. S., & Taylor, L. (2010). *Mental health in schools: Engaging learners, preventing problems, and improving schools*. Thousand Oaks, CA: Corwin.

Albee, G. W. (1989). No more rockscrubbing. *Journal of Community and Applied Social Psychology, 8*, 373–375.

Alpert-Gillis, L. J., Pedro-Carroll, J. L., & Cowen, E. L. (1989). The Children of Divorce Intervention Program: Development, implementation, and evaluation of a program for young urban children. *Journal of Consulting and Clinical Psychology, 57*, 583–589.

Alspaugh, J. (1998). Achievement loss associated with the transition to middle and high school. *Journal of Educational Research, 92*, 20–25.

Aos, D., Lieb, R., Mayfield, J. Miller, M., & Punnici, A. (2004). *Benefits and costs of prevention and early intervention programs for youth*. Olympia: Washington State Institute for Public Policy.

Banyard, V. L., & Goodman, L. (2009). Collaboration for building strong communities: Two examples. In M. E. Kenny, A. M. Horne, P. Orpinas, & L. E. Reese (Eds.), *Realizing social justice: The challenge of preventive interventions* (pp. 271–287). Washington, DC: American Psychological Association.

Barbarin, O. (2007). Mental health screening of preschool children: Validity and reliability of ABLE. *American Journal of Orthopsychiatry, 77,* 402–418.

Baskin, T. W., Slaten, C. D., Crosby, N. R., Pufahl, T., Schneller, C. L., & Ladell, M. (2010). Efficacy of counseling and psychotherapy in the schools: A meta-analytic review of treatment outcome studies. *The Counseling Psychologist, 38,* 878–903.

Beardslee, W. R., & Podorefsky, D. (1988). Resilient adolescents whose parents have serious affective and other psychiatric disorders: The importance of self-understanding and relationships. *American Journal of Psychiatry, 145,* 63–69.

Beauchamp, D. E. (1976). Public health as social justice. *Inquiry, 13,* 1–14.

Bellmore, A., & Graham, S. (2009). Disseminating scholarship to diverse audiences. In L. M. Dinella (Ed.), *Conducting science-based psychology research in schools* (pp. 199–214). Washington, DC: American Psychological Association.

Bergan, J. (1977). *Behavioral consultation.* Columbus, OH: Merrill.

Berkowitz, B., & Wolff, T. (2000). *The spirit of the coalition.* Washington, DC: American Public Health Association.

Biederman, J., Rosenbaum, J. F., Bolduc-Murphy, E. A., Faraone, S. V., Chaloff, J., Hirshfield, D. R., & Kagan, J. (1993). A 3-year follow-up study of children with and without behavioral inhibition. *Journal of the American Academy of Child and Adolescent Psychiatry, 32,* 814–821.

Bolger, K., & Patterson, C. (2003). Sequelae of child maltreatment. In S. S. Luthar (Ed.), *Resilience and vulnerability: Adaptation in the context of childhood adversities* (pp. 156–181). New York: Cambridge University Press.

Botvin, G. J. (2000). Preventing drug abuse in schools: Social and competence enhancement approaches targeting individual level etiological factors. *Addictive Behaviors, 25,* 887–897.

Botvin, G. J., & Kantor, L. W. (2000). Preventing alcohol and tobacco use through LifeSkills Training. *Alcohol Research and Health, 24,* 250–257.

Bradshaw, C. P., Koth, K., Bevans, K. B., Ialongo, N., & Leaf, P. J. (2008). The impact of school-wide positive behavioral interventions and supports on the organizational health of elementary schools. *School Psychology Quarterly, 23*, 462–473.

Brehm, K., & Doll, B. (2009). Building resilience in schools: A focus on population-based prevention. In R. W. Christner & R. B. Mennuti (Eds.), *School-based mental health: A practitioner's guide to comparative practices* (pp. 55–85). New York: Routledge.

Bronfenbrenner, U. (1979). *The ecology of human development.* Cambridge, MA: Harvard University Press.

Bullis, M., & Cheney, D. (1999). Vocational and transition interventions for adolescents and young adults with emotional or behavioral disorders. *Focus on Exceptional Children, 31*, 1–24.

Burns, B. J., Costello, E. J., Angold, A., Tweed, D., Stangl, D., Farmer, E. M., et al. (1995). Children's mental health service use across service sectors. *Health Affairs, 14*(3), 148–159.

Burns, M. K., & Gibbons, K. (2008). *Response to intervention implementation in elementary and secondary schools: Procedures to assure scientific-based practices.* New York: Routledge.

Carson, R. R., Sitlington, P. L., & Frank, A. R. (1995). Young adulthood for individuals with behavioral disorders: What does it hold? *Behavioral Disorders, 20,* 127–135.

Catalano, R. F., Berglund, M. L., Ryan, J. A. M., Lonczak, H. S., & Hawkins, J. D. (2004). Positive youth development in the United States: Research findings on evaluations of positive youth development programs. *Annals of the American Academy of Political and Social Science, 591*, 98–124.

Cattaneo, L. B., & Chapman, A. R. (2010). The process of empowerment. *American Psychologist, 65,* 646–659.

Centers for Disease Control and Prevention. (n.d.). *School Health Index.* Retrieved from http://www.cdc.gov/HealthyYouth/shi/

Centers for Disease Control and Prevention. (n.d.). *Youth Risk Behavior Surveillance System.* Retrieved from http://www.cdc.gov/HealthyYouth/yrbs/index.htm

Cicchetti, D. (2010). Developmental psychopathology. In M. E. Lamb, A. M. Freund, & R. M. Lerner (Eds.), *The handbook of life-span development: Vol. 2. Social and emotional development* (pp. 511–589). Hoboken, NJ: Wiley.

Cicchetti, D., & Rogosch, F. A. (1996). Equifinality and multifinality in developmental psychopathology. *Development and Psychopathology, 8*, 597–600.

Clarke, G. N., Hawkins, W. E., Murphy, M., Sheeber, L. B., Lewinsohn, P. M., & Seeley, J. R. (1995). Targeted prevention of unipolar depressive disorder in an at-risk sample of high school adolescents: A randomized trial of a group cognitive intervention. *Journal of the American Academy of Child and Adolescent Psychiatry, 34*, 312–321.

Clarke, G. N., Hornbrook, M., Lynch, F., Polen, M., Gale, J., Beardslee, W., et al. (2001). A randomized trial of a group cognitive intervention for preventing depression in adolescent offspring of depressed parents. *Archives of General Psychiatry, 58*, 1127–1134.

Cohen, L., & Swift, S. (1999). The spectrum of prevention: Developing a comprehensive approach to injury prevention. *Injury Prevention, 5*, 203–207.

Cohen, P., Brook, J. S., Cohen, J., Velez, C. N., & Garcia, M. (1990). Common and uncommon pathways to adolescent psychopathology and problem behavior. In L. N. Robins & M. Rutter (Eds.), *Straight and devious pathways from childhood* (pp. 242–258). New York: Cambridge University Press.

Coie, J. D., Watt, N. F., West, S. G., Hawkins, J. D., Asarnow, J. R., Markman, H. J., et al. (1993). The science of prevention: A conceptual framework and some directions for a national research program. *American Psychologist, 48*, 1013–1022.

Committee for Children. (2010). *Second Step.* Retrieved March 20, 2010, from http://www.cfchildren.org/programs/ssp/overview

Conduct Problems Prevention Research Group. (1999). Initial impact of the Fast Track prevention trial for conduct problems: I. The high-risk sample. *Journal of Consulting and Clinical Psychology, 67*, 631–647.

Cosner, S. (2009). Building organizational capacity through trust. *Educational Administration Quarterly, 45*, 248–291.

Costello, E. J., Angold, A., Burns, B. J., Stangl, D. K., Tweed, D. L., Erkanli, A., & Worthman, C. M. (1996). The Great Smoky Mountains Study of Youth: Functional impairment and severe emotional disturbance. *Archives of General Psychiatry, 53*, 1129–1136.

Costello, E. J., Foley, D. L., & Angold, A. (2006). 10-year research update review: The epidemiology of child and adolescent psychiatric disorders: II. *Journal of American Academy of Child and Adolescent Psychiatry, 45*, 8–25.

Costello, E. J., Messer, S. C., Bird, H. R., Cohen, P., & Reinherz, H. Z. (1998). The prevalence of serious emotional disturbance:

A re-analysis of community studies. *Journal of Children and Family Studies, 7,* 411–432.

Costello, E. J., Mustillo, S., Keeler, G., & Angold, A. (2004). Prevalence of psychiatric disorders in childhood and adolescence. In B. L. Levin, J. Petrila, & K. D. Hennessy (Eds.), *Mental health services: A public health perspective* (pp. 111–128). New York: Oxford University Press.

Cowen, E. L. (1973). Social and community interventions. *Annual Review of Psychology, 24,* 423–472.

Cowen, E. L. (1991). In pursuit of wellness. *American Psychologist, 46,* 404–408.

Cowen, E. L. (2000). Psychological wellness: Some hopes for the future. In D. Cicchetti, J. Rappaport, I. N. Sandler, & R. P. Weissberg (Eds.), *The promotion of wellness in children and adolescents* (pp. 477–503). Washington, DC: Child Welfare League of America.

Cowen, E. L., Hightower, A. D., Pedro-Carroll, J. L., Work, W. C., Wyman, P. A., & Haffey, W. G. (1996). *School-based prevention for children at risk: The primary mental health project.* Washington, DC: American Psychological Association.

Cowen, E. L., & Kilmer, R. P. (2002). "Positive psychology": Some plusses and some open issues (Commentary). *Journal of Community Psychology, 30,* 449–460. doi:10.1002/jcop.10014

Crews, S. D., Bender, H., Cook, C. R., Gresham, F. M., Kern, L., & Vanderwood, M. (2007). Risk and protective factors of emotional and/or behavioral disorders in children and adolescents: A mega-analytic synthesis. *Behavioral Disorders, 32*(2), 64–77.

Crick, N. R., Ostrov, J. M., Burr, J. E., Cullerton-Sen, C., Jansen-Yeh, E., & Ralston, P. (2006). A longitudinal study of relational and physical aggression in preschool. *Journal of Applied Developmental Psychology, 27,* 254–268.

Cuijpers, P., van Straten, A., Smit, F., Mihalopoulos, C., & Beekman, A. (2008). Preventing the onset of depressive disorders: A meta-analytic review of psychological interventions. *American Journal of Psychiatry, 165,* 1272–1280.

Cummings, J. A., Harrison, P. L., Dawson, M., Short, R. J., Gorin, S., & Palomares, R. S. (2004). Follow-up to the 2002 Futures Conference: Collaborating to serve all children, families, and schools. *Journal of Educational and Psychological Consultation, 15,* 335–344.

Curtis, M. J., Chesno Grier, J. E., & Hunley, S. A. (2003). The changing face of school psychology: Trends in data and projections for the future. *School Psychology Quarterly, 18*, 409–430.

Darling-Hammond, L., & Richardson, N. (2009). Teacher learning: What matters? *Educational Leadership, 66*(5), 46–53.

Datnow, A., & Stringfield, S. (2000). Working together for reliable school reform. *Journal for the Education of Students Placed at Risk, 5*, 183–204.

Davies, P. T., Sturge-Apple, M. L., Cicchetti, D., & Cummings, E. M. (2007). The role of child adrenocortical functioning in pathways between interparental conflict and child maladjustment. *Developmental Psychology, 43*, 918–930.

Dawson, M., Cummings, J. A., Harrison, P. L., Short, R. J., Gorin, S., & Palomares, R. (2004). The 2002 Multisite Conference on the Future of School Psychology: Next steps. *School Psychology Review, 33*, 115–125.

Deater-Deckard, K., & Dodge, K. A. (1997). Externalizing behavior problems and discipline revisited: Nonlinear effects and variation by culture, context, and gender. *Psychological Inquiry, 8*, 161–175.

de Voursney, D., Mannix, D., Brounstein, P. J., & Blau, G. M. (2008). Childhood growth and development. In T. P. Gullotta & G. M. Blau (Eds.), *Handbook of childhood behavioral issues: Evidence-based approaches to prevention and treatment* (pp. 19–39). New York: Routledge.

Doll, B., & Lyon, M. (1998). Risk and resilience: Implications for the delivery of educational and mental health services in schools. *School Psychology Review, 27*, 348–363.

Doll, B., & Yoon, J. (2010). The current status of youth prevention science. In B. Doll, W. Pfohl, & J Yoon (Eds.), *Handbook of youth prevention science* (pp. 1–18). New York: Routledge.

Domitrovich, C. E., Bradshaw, C. P., Greenberg, M. T., Embry, D., Poduska, J. M., & Ialongo, N. S. (2010). Integrated models of school-based prevention: Logic and theory. *Psychology in the Schools, 47*, 71–88.

Dowrick, P. W. (1998). A consideration of "community response programmes" for disabilities or other issues of common concern. *New Zealand Journal of Psychology, 27*(2), 30–35.

Dowrick, P. W., Power, T. J., Manz, P. H., Ginsburg-Block, M., Leff, S. Stephen, S., & Kim-Rupnow, S. (2001). Community responsiveness: Examples from under-resourced urban schools. *Journal of Prevention and Intervention in the Community, 21,* 71–90.

Drabick, D. A. G., & Kendall, P. C. (2010). Developmental psychopathology and the diagnosis of mental health problems among youth. *Clinical Psychology: Science and Practice, 17,* 272–280.

Dunst, C. J., Trivette, C. M., & Johanson, C. (1994). Parent-professional collaboration and partnerships. In C. J. Dunst, C. M. Trivette, & A. G. Deal (Eds.), *Supporting and strengthening families: Vol. 1. Methods, strategies and practices* (pp. 197–211). Cambridge, MA: Brookline Books.

Durlak, J. A. (1995). *School-based prevention programs for children and adolescents.* Thousand Oaks, CA: Sage.

Durlak, J. A. (1997). *Successful prevention programs for children and adolescents.* New York: Plenum.

Durlak, J. A., Taylor, R. D., Kawashima, K., Pachan, M. K., Du Pre, E. P., Celio, C. I., et al. (2007). Effects of positive youth development programs on school, family, and community systems. *American Journal of Community Psychology, 39,* 269–286.

Durlak, J. A., & Wells, A. M. (1997). Primary prevention mental health programs for children and adolescents: A meta-analytic review. *American Journal of Community Psychology, 25,* 115–152.

Eaton, D. K., Kann, L., Kinchen, S., Shanklin, S., Ross, J., Hawkins, J., et al. (2010). Youth risk behavior surveillance—United States, 2009. *Morbidity and Mortality Weekly Report, 59* (SS-5, June 4). Retrieved November 28, 2011 from http://www.cdc.gov/mmwr/pdf/ss/ss5905.pdf

Eber, L., & Nelson, C. M. (1997). Integrating services for students with emotional and behavioral needs through school-based wraparound planning. *American Journal of Orthopsychiatry, 67,* 385–395.

Eber, L., Sugai, G., Smith, C. R., & Scott, T. M. (2002). Wraparound and positive behavioral interventions and supports in the schools. *Journal of Emotional & Behavioral Disorders, 10,* 171–180.

Eccles, J., & Appleton, A. (Eds.). (2002). *Community programs to promote youth development.* Washington, DC: National Academies Press.

Egger, H. L., & Angold, A. (2006). Common emotional and behavioral disorders in preschool children: Presentation, nosology, and epidemiology. *Journal of Child Psychology and Psychiatry, 47*, 313–337.

Elias, M. J., Bruene-Butler, L., Bruno, E. M., Papke, M. R., & Shapiro, T. F. (2005). *SDM/SPS Social Decision Making/Social Problem Solving: A curriculum for academic, social, and emotional learning (Grades 4–5).* Champaign, IL: Research Press.

Elias, M. J., Gara, M., Ubriaco, M., & Rothbaum, P. A. (1986). Impact of a preventive social problem solving intervention on children's coping with middle-school stressors. *American Journal of Community Psychology, 14*, 259–275.

Elliott, S. N., & Busse, R. T. (2004). Assessment and evaluation of students' behavior and intervention outcomes: The utility of rating scale methods. In R. B. Rutherford, M. M. Quinn, & S. P. Mathur (Eds.), *Handbook of research in emotional and behavioral disorders* (pp. 123–142). New York: Guilford Press.

Embry, D. D., Staatemeier, G., Richardson, C., Lauger, K., & Mitich, J. (2003). *The PAX Good Behavior Game.* Center City, MN: Hazelden.

Ennett, S. T., Ringwalt, C. L., Thorne, J., Rohrback, L. A., Vincus, A., Simons-Rudolph, A., & Jones, S. (2003). A comparison of current practice in school-based substance use prevention programs with meta-analysis findings. *Prevention Science, 4*, 1–14.

Fetterman, D. M., & Wandersman, A. (2005). *Empowerment evaluation in practice.* New York: Guilford Press.

Frechtling, J. A. (2007). Logic modeling methods in program evaluation. San Francisco: Wiley.

Friedman, R. M., Best, K. A., Armstrong, M. I., Duchnowski, A. J., Evans, M. E., Hernandez, M., et al. (2004). Child mental health policy. In B. L. Levin, J. Petrila, & K. D. Hennessy (Eds.), *Mental health services: A public health perspective* (pp. 129–153). New York: Oxford University Press.

Friedman, R. M., Katz-Leavy, J. W., Manderscheid, R. W., & Sondheimer, D. (1996). Prevalence of serious emotional disturbance in children and adolescents. In R. W. Manderscheid & M. A. Sonnenschein (Eds.), *Mental Health, United States, 1996* (pp. 71–89). Rockville, MD: Center for Mental Health Services.

Friesen, B. J., & Stephens, B. (1998). Expanding family roles in the System of Care: Research and practice. In M. H.

Epstein, K. Kutash, & A. Duchnowski (Eds.), *Outcomes for children and youth with emotional and behavioral disorders and their families: Programs and evaluation best practices* (pp. 231–259). Austin, TX: PRO-ED.

Fullan, M., & Stiegelbauer, S. (1991). *The new meaning of educational change* (2nd ed.). New York: Teachers College Press.

Garland, A. F., Hough, R. L., McCabe, K. M., Yeh, M., Wood, P. A., & Aarons, G. A. (2001). Prevalence of psychiatric disorders across five sectors of care. *Journal of the American Academy of Child and Adolescent Psychiatry, 40*, 409–418.

Gibelman, M., & Kraft, S. (1996). Advocacy as a core agency program: Planning considerations for voluntary human service agencies. *Administration in Social Work, 20*(4), 43–59.

Gilman, R., Huebner, E. S., & Furlong, M. J. (2009). *Handbook of positive psychology in schools.* New York: Routledge.

Gordon, E. W. (2003). Urban education. *Teachers College Record, 105*, 189–207.

Gordon, R. (1987). An operational classification of disease prevention. In J. Steinberg & M. Silverman (Eds.), *Preventing mental disorders: A research perspective* (pp. 20–26). Rockville, MD: Department of Health and Human Services.

Grant, K. E., Compas, B. E., Thurm, A. E., McMahon, S. D., Gipson, P. Y., & Campbell, A. J. (2006). Stressors and child and adolescent psychopathology: Evidence of moderating and mediating effects. *Clinical Psychology Reviews, 26*, 257–283.

Graves, K. N., & Shelton, T. L. (2007). Family empowerment as a mediator between family-centered systems of care and changes in child functioning: Identifying an important mechanism of change. *Journal of Child and Family Studies, 16*, 556–566.

Greenberg, M. T., Domitrovich, C., & Bumbarger, B. (2001). The prevention of mental disorders in school-aged children: Current state of the field. *Prevention and Treatment, 4.*

Greenberg, M. T., & Kusché, C. A. (2006). Building social and emotional competence: The PATHS curriculum. In S. R. Jimerson & M. J. Furlong (Eds.), *Handbook of school violence and school safety: From research to practice* (pp. 395–412). Mahwah, NJ: Erlbaum.

Greenberg, M. T., Weissberg, R. P., O'Brien, M. U., Zins, J. E., Fredericks, L., Resnick, H., et al. (2003). Enhancing school-based prevention and youth development through coordinated social, emotional, and academic learning. *American Psychologist, 58*, 466–474.

Gresham, F. X., & Elliott, S N. (2008). *Social Skills Improvement System: Rating Scales.* Bloomington, MN: Pearson Assessments.

Gresham, F. X., Elliott, S. N., Vance, M. J., & Cook, C. R. (2011). Comparability of the Social Skills Rating System to the Social Skills Improvement System: Content and psychometric comparisons across elementary and secondary age levels. *School Psychology Quarterly, 26,* 27–44.

Groark, C., & McCall, R. B. (2005). Integrating developmental scholarship into practice and policy. In M. J. Bornstein & M. A. Lamb (Eds.), *Developmental science: An advanced textbook* (5th ed., pp. 557–601). Mahwah, NJ: Erlbaum.

Hall, G. E., & Hord, S. M. (2011). *Implementing change: Patterns, principles, and potholes* (3rd ed.). Boston: Pearson.

Hawkins, J. D., Catalano, R. F., & Miller, J. Y. (1992). Risk and protective factors for alcohol and other drug problems in adolescent and early adulthood: Implications for substance abuse prevention. *Psychological Bulletin, 112,* 64–105.

Henggeler, S. W., & Lee, T. (2003). Multisystemic treatment of serious clinical problems. In A. E. Kazdin & J. R. Weisz (Eds.), *Evidence-based psychotherapies for children and adolescents* (pp. 301–322). New York: Guilford Press.

Henggeler, S. W., Schoenwald, S. K., Rowland, M. D., & Cunningham, P. B. (2002). *Serious emotional disturbance in children and adolescents: Multisystemic Therapy.* New York: Guilford Press.

Hightower, A. D., Johnson, D., & Haffey, W. G. (1995). Best practices in adopting a prevention program. In A. Thomas & J. Grimes (Eds.), *Best practices in school psychology* (3rd ed., pp. 311–323).Washington, DC: National Association of School Psychologists.

Hoagwood, K., Burns, B. J., & Weisz, J. R. (2002). A profitable conjunction: From science to service in Children's Mental Health. In B. J. Burns, & K. Hoagwood (Eds.), *Community treatment for youth: Evidence-based interventions for severe emotional and behavioral disorders* (pp. 1079–1089). New York: Oxford University Press.

Hoagwood, K., & Johnson, J. (2003). School psychology: A public health framework. I. From evidence-based practices to evidence-based policies. *Journal of School Psychology, 41,* 3–21.

Hoefer, R. (2006). *Advocacy practice for social justice.* Chicago: Lyceum.

Horner, R. H., Sugai, G., Todd, A. W., & Lewis-Palmer, T. (2005). School-wide positive behavior support. In L. Bambara & L. Kern (Eds.), *Individualized supports for students with problem behaviors: Designing positive behavior plans* (pp. 359–390). New York: Guilford Press.

Horowitz, J. L., & Garber, J. (2006). The prevention of depressive symptoms in children and adolescents: A meta-analytic review. *Journal of Consulting and Clinical Psychology, 74,* 401–415.

Horsch, K. (1997). *Indicators: Definition and use in a results-based accountability system.* Cambridge, MA: Harvard Family Research Project. Retrieved from http://www.hfrp.org/publications-resources/browse-our-publications/indicators-definition-and-use-in-a-results-based-accountability-system

Ialongo, N. S., Rogosch, F. A., Cicchetti, D., Toth, S. L., Buckley, J., Petras, H., et al. (2006). A developmental psychopathology approach to the prevention of health disorders. In D. Cicchetti & D. J. Cohen (Eds.), *Developmental psychopathology: Vol. 1. Theory and method* (2nd ed., pp. 968–1018). Hoboken, NJ: Wiley.

Institute of Medicine. (1988). *The future of public health.* Washington, DC: National Academy Press.

Institute of Medicine, Committee on Prevention of Mental Disorders. (1994). *Reducing risks for mental disorders mental disorders: Frontiers for preventive intervention research* (P. J. Mrazek & R. J. Haggerty, Eds.). Washington, DC: National Academy Press.

Joint Commission on Mental Health of Children. (1970). *Crisis in child mental health: Challenge for the 1970s.* New York: Harper & Row.

Kataoka, S. H., Zhang, L., & Wells, K. B. (2002). Unmet need for mental health care among U.S. children: Variation by ethnicity and insurance status. *American Journal of Psychiatry, 159,* 1548–1555.

Kellam, S. G., & Langevin, D. J. (2003). A framework for understanding "evidence" in prevention research and programs. *Prevention Science, 4,* 137–153.

Kenny, M. E., Horne, A. M., Orpinas, P., & Reese, L. E. (2009). Social justice and the challenge of preventive interventions: An introduction. In M. E. Kenny, A. M. Horne, P. Orpinas, & L. E. Reese (Eds.), *Realizing social justice: The challenge of preventive interventions* (pp. 17–35). Washington, DC: American Psychological Association.

Kern, L., Hilt-Panahon, A., & Sokol, N. G. (2009). Further examining the triangle tip: Improving support for students with emotional and behavioral needs. *Psychology in the Schools, 46*, 18–32.

Kessler, R. C., Berglund, P., Demler, P., Jin, R., Merikangas, K. R., & Walters, E. E. (2005). Lifetime prevalence and age-of-onset distributions of DSM-IV disorders in the national comorbidity survey replication. *Archives of General Psychiatry, 62*, 593–602.

Kessler, R. C., Foster, C. L., Saunders, W. B., & Stang, P. E. (1995). Social consequences of psychiatric disorders, I: Educational attainment. *American Journal of Psychiatry, 152*, 1026–1032.

Keys, S. G., & Leaf, P. H. (2008). Public health principles and approaches to systems interventions to support children's emotional and behavioral health. In T. P. Gullotta & G. M. Blau (Eds.), *Family influences on childhood behavior and development: Evidence-based prevention and treatment approaches* (pp. 97–116). New York: Routledge.

Kirkwood, A. D., & Stamm, B. H. (2006). A social marketing approach to challenging stigma. *Professional Psychology: Research and Practice, 37*(5), 472–476.

Kotler, P., & Roberto, E. (1989). *Social marketing: Strategies for changing public behavior.* New York: Free Press.

Knitzer, J. (2005). Advocacy for children's mental health: A personal journey. *Journal of Clinical Child and Adolescent Psychology, 34*(4), 612–618.

Knitzer, J. E. (1976). Child advocacy: A perspective. *Annual Progress in Child Psychiatry and Child Development, 47*, 372–373.

Knowlton, L. W., & Phillips, C. C. (2009). *The logic model guidebook: Better strategies for great results.* Los Angeles: Sage.

Kraemer, H. C., Kazdin, A. E., Offord, D. R., Kessler, R. C., Jensen, P. S., & Kupfer, D. (1997). Coming to terms with the terms of risk. *Archives of General Psychiatry, 54*, 337–343.

Krieger, N. (2001). A glossary for social epidemiology. *Journal of Epidemiology and Community Health, 55*, 693–700.

Kusché, C. A., & Greenberg, M. T. (1994). *The PATHS (Promoting Alternative Thinking Strategies) curriculum.* Deerfield, MA: Channing-Bete.

Lassen, S. R., Steele, M. M., & Sailor, W. (2006). The relationship of school-wide positive behavior support to academic achievement in an urban middle school. *Psychology in the Schools, 43*, 701–712.

Last, J. M. (1988). *A dictionary of epidemiology* (2nd ed.). New York: Oxford University Press.

Lawson, H. A. (2003). Pursuing and securing collaboration to improve results. In M. M. Brabeck, M. E. Walsh, & R. E. Latta (Eds.), *Meeting at the hyphen: Schools-universities-communities-professions in collaboration for student achievement and well being* (pp. 45–73). Chicago: University of Chicago Press.

Leadbeater, B. J., Schellenbach, C. J., Maton, K. I., & Dodgen, D. W. (2004). Research and policy for building strengths: Processes and contexts of individual, family, and community development. In K. I. Maton, C. J. Schellenbach, B. J. Leadbeater, & A . L. Solarz (Eds.), *Investing in children, youth, families, and communities: Strengths-based research and policy* (pp. 13–30). Washington, DC: American Psychological Association.

Levine, M., Perkins, D. D., & Perkins, D. V. (2005). *Prevention. Principles of community psychology: Perspectives and applications* (3rd ed., pp. 271–325). New York: Oxford University Press.

Levitt, J., Saka, N., Romanelli, L., & Hoagwood, K. (2007). Early identification of mental health problems in schools: The status of instrumentation. *Journal of School Psychology 45*, 163–191.

Lloyd, J. W., Kauffman, J. M., Landrum, T. J., & Roe, D. L. (1991). Why do teachers refer pupils for special education? An analysis of referral records. *Exceptionality, 2*(3), 115–126.

Lochman, J. E., & Wells, K. C. (2002). The Coping Power program at the middle school transition universal and indicated prevention effects. *Psychology of Addictive Behaviors, 16*(4 Suppl.), S40–S54.

Lochman, J. E., Wells, K. C., & Lenhart, L. A. (2008). *Coping Power: Child group program, facilitator's manual.* Programs ThatWork™. New York: Oxford University Press.

Luthar, S. S. (2006). Resilience in development: A synthesis of research across five decades. In D. Cicchetti & D. J. Cohen (Eds.), *Developmental psychopathology: Vol. 3. Risk, disorder, and adaptation* (2nd ed., pp. 739–795). New York: Wiley.

Luthar, S. S., Cicchetti, D., Becker, B. (2000). The construct of resilience: A critical evaluation and guidelines for future work. *Child Development, 71,* 543–562.

Lyman, D. R., Milich, R., Simmerman, R., Novak, S. P., Logan, T. K., Martin, C., et al. (1999). Project DARE: No effects at 10-year follow-up. *Journal of Consulting and Clinical Psychology, 67,* 590–593.

Ma, L., Phelps, E., Lerner, J. V., & Lerner, R. M. (2009). The development of academic competence among adolescents who bully and who are bullied. *Journal of Applied Developmental Psychology, 30,* 628–644.

MacMillan, H. L., Fleming, J. E., Streiner, D. L., Lin, E., Boyle, M. H., & Jamieson, E. (2001). Childhood abuse and lifetime psychopathology in a community sample. *American Journal of Psychiatry, 158,* 1878–1883.

Malloy, J., Cheney, D., & Cormier, G. (1998). Interagency collaboration and the transition to adulthood for students with emotional or behavioral disabilities. *Education and Treatment of Children, 1,* 303–320.

Masten, A. S. (2001). Ordinary magic: Resilience processes in development. *American Psychologist, 56,* 227–238.

Maton, K. (2008). Empowering community settings: Agents of individual development, community betterment, and positive social change. *American Journal of Community Psychology, 41,* 4–21.

Maton, K. I., Schellenbach, C. J., Leadbeater, B. J., & Solarz, A. L. (2004). *Investing in children, youth, families, and communities.* Washington, DC: American Psychological Association.

Mayes, L. C., & Suchman, N. (2006). Developmental pathways to substance abuse. In D. Cicchetti & D. Cohen (Eds.), *Developmental psychopathology: Risk, disorder, and adaptation* (Vol. 3, pp. 599–619). New York: Wiley.

McConaughy, S. H., & Leone, P. E. (2002). Measuring the success of prevention programs. In B. Algozzine & P. Kay (Eds.), *Preventing problem behaviors* (pp. 183–219). Thousand Oaks, CA: Corwin.

McKay, M., Jensen, P. S., & CHAMPS Collaborative Board. (2010). Collaborating with consumers, providers, systems and communities to enhance child mental health services research. In K E. Hoagwood, P. S. Jensen, M. McKay, & S. Olin (Eds.), *Children's mental health research: The power of partnerships* (pp. 14–39). New York: Oxford University Press.

McMahon, S. D., Grant, K. E., Compas, B. E., Thurm, A. E., & Ey, S. (2003). Stress and psychopathology in children and adolescents: Is there evidence of specificity? *Journal of Child Psychology and Psychiatry and the Allied Disciplines: Annual Research Review, 44*, 107–133.

McMahon, T., Ward, N., Pruett, M., Davidson, L., & Griffith, E. (2000). Building full-service schools: Lessons learned in the development of interagency collaboratives. *Journal of Educational and Psychological Consultation, 11*, 65–92.

McQuillan, P. J. (2005). Possibilities and pitfalls: A comparative analysis of student empowerment. *American Educational Research Journal, 42*, 639–670.

Mead, M. (n.d.). *BrainyQuote.com.* Retrieved March 22, 2011, from BrainyQuote.com Web site: http://www.brainyquote.com/quotes/authors/m/margaret_mead.html

Melhem, N. M., Walker, M., Moritz, G., & Brent, D. A. (2008). Antecedents and sequelae of sudden parental death in offspring and surviving caregivers. *Archives of Pediatrics and Adolescent Medicine, 162*, 403–410.

Melton, G. B. (2005). Treating children like people: A framework for research and advocacy. *Journal of Clinical Child and Adolescent Psychology, 34*, 646–657.

Merriam-Webster's Collegiate Dictionary (11th ed.). (2008). "Problem." Springfield, MA: Merriam-Webster.

Merrill, K. W., & Buchanan, R. (2006). Intervention selection in school-based practice: Using public health models of enhance systems capacity of schools. *School Psychology Review, 35*, 167–180.

Meyers, J. (2002). A 30-year perspective on best practices for consultation training. *Journal of Educational and Psychological Consultation, 13*, 35–54.

Miles, J., Espiritu, R.C., Horen, N., Sebian, J., & Waetzig, E. (2010). *A public health approach to children's mental health: A conceptual framework.* Washington, DC: Georgetown University Center for Child and Human Development, National Technical Assistance Center for Children's Mental Health.

Miltenberger, R. G. (2008). *Behavior modification: Principles and procedures* (4th ed.). Belmont, CA: Wadsworth.

Molgaard, V., & Spoth, R. (2001). The Strengthening Families Program for young adolescents: Overview and outcomes. In S. Pfeiffer & L. Reddy (Eds.), *Innovative mental health interventions for children: Programs that work* (pp. 15–29). Binghamton, NY: Haworth Press.

Nastasi, B. K. (2004). Meeting the challenges of the future: Integrating public health and public education for mental health promotion. *Journal of Educational and Psychological Consultation, 15,* 295–312.

Nastasi, B. K., Moore, R. B., & Varjas, K. M. (2004). *School-based mental health services: Creating comprehensive and culturally specific programs.* Washington, DC: American Psychological Association.

Nastasi, B. K., Varjas, K., Schensul, S. L., Silva, K. T., Schensul, J. J., & Ratnayake, P. (2000). The Participatory Intervention Model: A framework for conceptualizing and promoting intervention acceptability. *School Psychology Quarterly, 15,* 207–232.

National Association of School Psychologists. (2010). *Model of Comprehensive and Integrated School Psychological Services.* Retrieved from http://www.nasponline.org/standards/2010standards/2_PracticeModel.pdf

National Research Council & Institute of Medicine. (1988). *The future of public health.* Committee for the Study of the Future of Public Health, Division of Health Care Services. Washington, DC: National Academies Press.

National Research Council & Institute of Medicine. (2004). *Children's health, the nation's wealth: Assessing and improving children's health.* Committee on Evaluation of Children's Health, Board of Children, Youth, and Families, Division of Behavioral and Social Sciences and Education. Washington, DC: National Academies Press.

National Research Council & Institute of Medicine. (2009). *Preventing mental, emotional, and behavioral disorders among young people: Progress and possibilities* (M. E. O'Connell, T. Boat, & K. E. Warner, Eds.). Committee on the Prevention of Mental Disorders and Substance Abuse Among Children, Youth, and Young Adults: Research Advances and Promising Interventions. Washington, DC: National Academies Press.

Nelson, G., Prilleltensky, I., & MacGillivary, H. (2001). Building value-based partnerships: Toward solidarity with oppressed groups. *American Journal of Community Psychology, 29*(5), 649–677.

Nix, R. L., Pinderhughes, E. E., Bierman, K. L., Maples, J. J., & Conduct Problems Prevention Research Group. (2005). Decoupling the relation between risk factors for conduct problems and the receipt of intervention services:

Participation across multiple components of a prevention program. *American Journal of Community Psychology, 36,* 307–325.

O'Farrell, S. L., Morrison, G. M., & Furlong, M. J. (2006). School engagement. In G. G. Bear & K. M. Minke (Eds.), *Children's needs III: Development, prevention, and intervention* (pp. 45–58). Bethesda, MD: National Association of School Psychologists.

Pedro-Carroll, J. L., & Alpert-Gillis, L. J. (1997). Preventive interventions for children of divorce: A developmental model for 5 and 7 year old children. *Journal of Primary Prevention, 18,* 5–23.

Pedro-Carroll, J. L., & Cowen, E. L. (1987). The Children of Divorce Intervention Program: Implementation and evaluation of a time limited group approach. In J. Vincent (Ed.), *Advances in family intervention, assessment, and theory* (Vol. 4, 281–307). Greenwich, CT: JAI Press.

Pedro-Carroll, J. L., Cowen, E. L., Hightower, A. D., & Guare, J. C. (1986). Preventive intervention with latency-aged children of divorce: A replication study. *American Journal of Community Psychology, 14,* 277–289.

Perry, C. L., Williams, C. L., Forster, J. L., Wolfson, M., Wagenaar, A. C., Finnegan, J. R., et al. (1993). Background, conceptualization and design of a community-wide research program on adolescent alcohol use: Project Northland. *Health Education Research, 8,* 125–136.

Perry, C. L., Williams, C. L., Komro, K. A., Veblen-Mortenson, S., Forster, J. L., Bernstein-Lachter, R., et al. (2000). Project Northland high school interventions: Community action to reduce adolescent alcohol use. *Health Education and Behavior, 27,* 29–49.

Petras, H., Kellam, S. G., Brown, C. H., Muthen, B. O., Ialongo, N. S., & Poduska, J. M. (2008). Developmental epidemiological courses leading to antisocial personality disorder and violent and criminal behavior: Effects by young adulthood of a universal preventive intervention in first- and second-grade classrooms. *Drug and Alcohol Dependence, 95*(Suppl.1), 45–59.

Pina, A. A., Villalta, I. K., Ortiz, C. D., Gottschall, A. C., Costa, N. M., & Weems, C. F. (2008). Social support, discrimination, and coping as predictors of posttraumatic stress reactions in youth survivors of Hurricane Katrina. *Journal of Clinical Child and Adolescent Psychology, 37,* 564–574.

Power, T. J., Dowrick, P. W., Ginsburg-Block, M., & Manz, P. H. (2004). Partnership-based, community-assisted early intervention for literacy: An application of the Participatory Intervention Model. *Journal of Behavioral Education, 13,* 93–115.

Power, T. J., DuPaul, G. J., Shapiro, E. S., & Kazak, A. E. (2003). *Promoting children's health: Integrating school, family, and community.* New York: Guilford Press.

Prout, H. T., & DeMartino, R. A. (1986). A meta-analysis of school-based studies of counseling and psychotherapy. *Journal of School Psychology, 24,* 285–292.

Prout, S. M., & Prout, H. T. (1998). A meta-analysis of school-based studies of counseling and psychotherapy: An update. *Journal of School Psychology, 36,* 121–136.

Pumariega, A. J., & Winters, N. C. (Eds.). (2003). *The handbook of child and adolescent systems of care.* San Francisco: Jossey-Bass.

Raine, A., Brennan, P., & Mednick, S. A. (1997). Interaction between birth complications and early maternal rejection in predisposing individuals to adult violence: Specificity to serious, early-onset violence. *American Journal of Psychiatry, 154,* 1265-1271.

Ramey, C. T., & Ramey, S. L. (1998). Early intervention and early experience. *American Psychologist, 53,* 109–120.

Rappaport, J. (1987). Terms of empowerment/exemplars of prevention: Toward a theory for community psychology. *American Journal of Community Psychology, 15,* 121–148.

Reese, R. J., Prout, H. T., Zirkelback, E. A., & Anderson, C. R. (2010). Effectiveness of school-based psychotherapy: A meta-analysis of dissertation research. *Psychology in the Schools, 47,* 1035–1045.

Reschly, D. J., & Ysseldyke, J. E. (2002). Paradigm shift: The past is not the future. In A. Thomas & J. Grimes (Eds.), *Best practices in school psychology* (4th ed., pp. 3–20). Bethesda, MD: National Association of School Psychologists.

Resendez, M. G., Quist, R. M., & Matshazi, D. G. M. (2000). A longitudinal analysis of family empowerment and client outcomes. *Journal of Child and Family Studies, 9,* 449–460.

Robinson, K. E., & Rapport, L. J. (2002). Outcomes of a school-based mental health program for youth with serious emotional disorders. *Psychology in the Schools, 39,* 661–675.

Rogers, E. M. (1995). *Diffusion of innovations* (4th ed.). New York: Free Press.

Rogers, E. M. (2002). Diffusion of preventative innovations. *Addictive Behaviors, 27,* 989–993.

Roosa, M. W., Dumka, L. E., Gonzales, N. A., & Knight, G. P. (2002). Cultural/ethnic issues and the prevention scientist in the 21st century. *Prevention and Treatment, 5.*

Roosa, M. W., Sandler, I. N., Gehring, M., Beals, J., & Cappo, L. (1988). The Children of Alcoholics Life Events Schedule: A stress scale for children of alcohol abusing parents. *Journal of Studies on Alcohol, 49,* 422–429.

Rosenblatt, J. L., & Elias, M. J. (2008). Dosage effects of a preventive social-emotional learning intervention on achievement loss associated with middle school transition. *Journal of Primary Prevention, 29,* 535–555.

Rosenfield, S. (2008). Best practices in instructional consultation and instructional consultation teams. In A. Thomas & J. Grimes (Eds.), *Best practices in school psychology* (5th ed., pp. 1645–1660). Bethesda, MD: National Association of School Psychologists.

Ross, R. G., Radant, A. D., Heinlein, S., & Compagnon, N. (2003). Smooth pursuit eye movement abnormalities in children with and vulnerable to schizophrenia. *Schizophrenia Research, 60*(1), Suppl. 1, 268–269.

Rous, B., Myers, C. T., & Stricklin, S. B. (2007). Strategies for supporting transitions of young children with special needs and their families. *Journal of Early Intervention, 30,* 1–18.

Rutter, M. (1987). Psychosocial resilience and protective mechanisms. *American Journal of Orthopsychiatry, 57,* 316–331.

Rutter, M., & Maughan, B. (2002). School effectiveness findings 1979-2002. *Journal of School Psychology, 40,* 451–475.

Sallis, J. F., Owen, N., & Fotheringham, M. J. (2000). Behavioral epidemiology: A systematic framework to classify phases of research on health promotion and disease prevention. *Annals of Behavioral Medicine, 4,* 294–298.

Sandler, I. N., Wolchik, S. A., Braver, S. L., & Fogas, B. S. (1986). Significant events of children and divorce: Toward the assessment of a risky situation. In S. M. Auerbach & A. Stolberg (Eds.), *Crisis intervention with children and families* (pp. 65–83). New York: Hemisphere.

Scales, P. C., & Leffert, N. (1999). *Developmental assets: A synthesis of the scientific research on adolescent development.* Minneapolis, MN: Search Institute.

Scott, T. M., & Eber, L. (2003). Functional assessment and wrap-around as systemic school processes: Primary, secondary and tertiary systems examples. *Journal of Emotional and Behavioral Disorders, 5,* 131–143.

Segal, S., Silverman, C., & Temkin, T. (1995). Measuring empowerment in client-run self-help agencies. *Community Mental Health Journal, 31,* 215–227.

Seidman, E., Allen, L., Aber, J., & Mitchell, C. (1994). The impact of school transitions in early adolescence on the self-system and perceived social context of poor urban youth. *Child Development, 65,* 507–522.

Seligman, M. E. P., & Csikszentmihalyi, M. (2000). Happiness, excellence, and optimal human functioning [Special issue]. *American Psychologist, 55.*

Semple, D. M., McIntosh, A. M., & Lawrie, S. M. (2005). Cannabis as a risk factor for psychosis: Systematic review. *Journal of Psychopharmacology, 19,* 187–194.

Severson, H. H., Walker, H. M., Hope-Doolittle, J., Kratochwill, T. R., & Gresham, F. M. (2007). Proactive, early screening to detect behaviorally at-risk students: Issues, approaches, emerging innovations, and professional practices. *Journal of School Psychology, 45,* 193–223.

Shankman, S. A., Lewinsohn, P. M., Klein, D. N., Small, J. W., Seeley, J. R., & Altman, S. E. (2009). Subthreshold conditions as precursors for full syndrome disorders: A 15-year longitudinal study of multiple diagnostic classes. *Journal of Child Psychology and Psychiatry, 50,* 1485–1494.

Shapiro, E. S. (2006). Are we solving the big problems? *School Psychology Review, 35,* 260–265.

Sheridan, S. M., & Gutkin, T. G. (2000). The ecology of school psychology: Examining and changing our paradigm for the 21st century. *School Psychology Review, 29,* 485–502.

Short, R. J., & Brokaw, R. (1994). Externalizing behavior disorders. In R. J. Simeonsson (Ed.), *Risk, resilience, and prevention: Promoting the well-being of all children* (pp. x–xx). Baltimore: Brookes.

Short, R. J., & Shapiro, S. K. (1993). Conduct disorders: A framework for understanding and intervention in schools and communities. *School Psychology Review, 22,* 362–375.

Short, R. J., & Strein, W. (2007). Social and behavioral epidemiology: Population-based problem identification and monitoring. In B. J. Doll & J. A. Cummings (Eds.), *Transforming school mental health services* (pp. 23–42). Bethesda, MD: National Association of School Psychologists.

Short, R. J., & Talley, R. C. (1999). Services integration: An introduction. *Journal of Educational and Psychological Consultation, 10,* 193–200.

Shriberg, D., Bonner, M., Sarr, B. J., Walker, A. M., Hyland, M., & Chester, C. (2008). Social justice through a school psychology lens: Definition and application. *School Psychology Review, 37,* 453–468.

Shure, M. B., & Spivack, G. (1988). Interpersonal cognitive problem solving. In R. H. Price, E. L. Cowen, R. P. Lorion, & J. Ramos-McKay (Eds.), *14 ounces of prevention: A casebook for practitioners* (pp. 69–82). Washington, DC: American Psychological Association.

Simeonsson, R. J. (1994). Toward an epidemiology of developmental, educational, and social problems of childhood. In R. J. Simeonsson (Ed.), *Risk, resilience & prevention: Promoting the well-being of all children.* (pp. 13–31). Baltimore: Brookes.

Simon, B. I. (1994). *The empowerment tradition in American social work: A history.* New York: Columbia University Press.

Slade, E. P. (2002). Effects of school-based mental health programs on mental health service use by adolescents at school and in the community. *Mental Health Services Research, 4,* 151–166.

Spoth, R., Greenberg, M., Bierman, K., & Redmond, C. (2004). PROSPER community–university partnership model for public education systems: Capacity-building for evidence-based, competence-building prevention. *Prevention Science, 5,* 31–39.

Stephens, R. D. (1998). Safe school planning. In D. S. Elliott, B. A. Hamburg, & K. R. Williams (Eds.), *Violence in American schools: A new perspective* (pp. 253–289). Cambridge, UK: Cambridge University Press.

Stroul, B. A., & Friedman, R. M. (1996). The System of Care concept and philosophy. In B. A. Stroul (Ed.), *Children's mental health: Creating systems of care in a changing society* (pp. 3–21). Baltimore: Brookes.

Sugai, G., & Horner, R. R. (2006). A promising approach for expanding and sustaining school-wide positive behavior support. *School Psychology Review, 35,* 245–259.

Sugai, G., & Horner, R. H. (2008). What we know and need to know about preventing problem behaviors in the schools. *Exceptionality, 16*, 67–77.

Sugai, G., Sprague, J. R., Horner, R. H., & Walker, H. M. (2000). Preventing school violence: The use of office discipline referrals to assess and monitor school-wide discipline interventions. *Journal of Emotional and Behavioral Disorders, 8*, 94–101.

Suter, J. C., & Bruns, E. J. (2009). Effectiveness of the wraparound process for children with emotional and behavioral disorders: A meta-analysis. *Clinical Child and Family Psychology Review, 12*, 336–351.

Telzrow, C. F., & Beebe, J. J. (2002). Best practices in facilitating intervention adherence and integrity. In A. Thomas and J. Grimes (Eds.), *Best practices in school psychology* (4th ed., pp. 503–516). Bethesda, MD: National Association of School Psychologists.

Thompson, L., Lobb, C., Elling, R., Herman, S., Jurkiewicz, T., & Hulleza, C. (1997). Pathways to family empowerment: Effects of family-centered delivery of early intervention services. *Exceptional Children, 64*, 99–113.

Tilly, D. W. (2002). Best practices in school psychology as a problem-solving enterprise. In A. Thomas & J. Grimes (Eds.), *Best practices in school psychology* (4th ed., pp. 21–36). Washington, DC: National Association of School Psychologists.

U.S. Department of Education. (2005). *Twenty-seventh annual report to Congress*. Washington, DC: Author.

U.S. Department of Health and Human Services. (1999). *Mental health: A report of the Surgeon General*. Rockville, MD: U.S. Public Health Service.

U.S. Department of Health and Human Services. (2001). *Mental health: Culture, race, and ethnicity: A report of the Surgeon General*. Rockville, MD: U.S. Public Health Service.

U.S. Public Health Service. (2000). *Report of the Surgeon General's conference on children's mental health: A nation action agenda*. Washington, DC: U.S. Department of Health and Human Services.

U.S. Public Health Service. (2001). *Youth violence: A report of the Surgeon General*. Washington, DC: Author.

Vanderploeg, J. J., Franks, R. P., Plant, R., Cloud, M., & Tebes, J. K. (2009). Extended Day Treatment: A comprehensive model of after school behavioral health services for youth. *Child and Youth Care Forum, 38*, 5–18.

Walker, H. M., Nishioka, V. M., Zeller, R., Severson, H. H., & Feil, E. G. (2000). Causal factors and potential solutions for the persistent under-identification of students having emotional or behavioral disorders in the context of schooling. *Assessment for Effective Intervention, 26*, 29–40.

Walker, H. M., Seeley, J. R., Small, J., Severson, H. H., Graham, B. A., Feil, E. G., et al. (2009). A randomized controlled trial of the First Step to Success early intervention: Demonstration of program efficacy outcomes in a diverse, urban school district. *Journal of Emotional and Behavioral Disorders, 17*, 197–212.

Walker, H. M., & Severson, H. H. (1990). *Systematic Screening for Behavior Disorders.* Longmont, CO: Sopris West.

Webb, P., Bain, C., & Pirozzo, S. (2005). *Essential epidemiology.* Cambridge, UK: Cambridge University Press.

Webster-Stratton, C. (1982). Teaching mothers through videotape modeling to change their children's behaviors. *Journal of Pediatric Psychology, 7*, 279–294.

Webster-Stratton, C., & Herman, K. C. (2010). Disseminating Incredible Years series early-intervention programs: Integrating and sustain services between school and home. *Psychology in the Schools, 47*, 36–54.

Weisz, J. R., Sandler, I. N., Durlak, J. A., & Anton, S. A. (2005). Promoting and protecting youth mental health through evidence-based prevention and treatment. *American Psychologist, 60*, 628–648.

Weiss, B., Catron, T., Harris, V., & Phung, T. M. (1999). The effectiveness of traditional child psychotherapy. *Journal of Clinical and Consulting Psychology, 67*, 82–94.

Weissberg, R. P., Kumpfer, K. L., & Seligman, M. E. P. (2003) Prevention that works for children and youth: An introduction. *American Psychologist, 58,* 425–432.

Weist, M. D., Ambrose, M. G., & Lewis, C. P. (2006). Expanded school mental health: A collaborative community example. *Children & Schools, 28*, 45–50.

Werner, E. (2006). What can we learn about resilience from large-scale longitudinal studies? In S. Goldstein & R. Brooks (Eds.), *Handbook of resilience in children* (pp. 91–105). New York: Springer.

Werner, E., & Smith, R. (1982). *Vulnerable but invincible: A study of resilient children.* New York: McGraw-Hill.

Wolfendale, S. (1992). *Empowering parents and teachers: Working for children.* London: Cassell.

World Health Organization. (2004). *Prevention of mental disorders: Effective interventions and policy options, Summary report*. A report of the World Health Organization in collaboration with the Prevention Research Centre of the University of Nijmegen and Maastrict. Geneva, Switzerland: Author. Retrieved from http://www.who.int/mental_health/evidence/en/prevention_of_mental_disorders_sr.pdf

World Health Organization. (2005). *Promoting mental health: concepts, emerging evidence, practice*. Retrieved from http://www.who.int/mental_health/evidence/MH_Promotion_Book.pdf

Wyman, P. A. (2003). Emerging perspectives on context specificity of children's adaptation and resilience: Evidence from a decade of research with urban children in adversity. In S. Luthar (Ed.), *Resilience and vulnerability: Adaptation in the context of childhood adversity* (pp. 293–317). New York: Cambridge University Press.

Ysseldyke, J., Burns, M., Dawson, P., Kelley, B., Morrison, D., Ortiz, S., et al. (2006). *School psychology: A blueprint for training and practice III. [Blueprint III]* Bethesda, MD: National Association of School Psychologists.

Ysseldyke, J., Burns, M., Dawson, P., Kelley, B., Morrison, D., Ortiz, S., et al. (2008). The blueprint for training and practice as the basis for best practices. In A. Thomas & J. Grimes (Eds.), *Best practices in school psychology V* (pp. 37–70). Bethesda, MD: National Association of School Psychologists.

Zigler, E., & Muenchow, S. (1992). *Head Start: The inside story of America's most successful educational experiment*. New York: Basic Books.

Zimmerman, M. A. (1995). Psychological empowerment: Issues and illustrations. *American Journal of Community Psychology, 32*, 581–599.

Zins, J. E., Weissberg, R. P., Wang, M. C., & Walberg, H. J. (Eds.). (2004). *Building academic success on social and emotional learning: What does the research say?* New York: Teachers College Press.

Index

CD Contents